ADVANCES IN THE BIOSCIENCES

Volume 88

CARDIOVASCULAR AND RENAL ACTIONS OF DOPAMINE

ADVANCES IN THE BIOSCIENCES

Latest volumes in the series:

CARDIOVASCULAR AND RENAL ACTIONS OF DOPAMINE

Proceedings of the IVth International Conference on Peripheral Dopamine held in Porto, Portugal on 18–20 June 1992

Editor:

P. SOARES-DA-SILVA

Department of Pharmacology and Therapeutics, Faculty of Medicine, University of Porto, 4200 Porto, Portugal

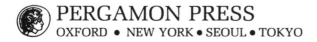 PERGAMON PRESS

OXFORD • NEW YORK • SEOUL • TOKYO

U.K.	Pergamon Press Ltd, Headington Hill Hall, Oxford OX3 0BW, England
U.S.A	Pergamon Press Inc., 660 White Plains Road, Tarrytown, New York 10591-5153, U.S.A.
KOREA	Pergamon Press Korea, Room 705 Hanaro Building, 194-4 Insa-Dong, Chongno-ku, Seoul 110-794, Korea
JAPAN	Pergamon Press, Tsunashima Building Annex, 3-20-12 Yushima, Bunkyo-ku, Tokyo 113, Japan

First edition 1993

ISBN: 0-08-042209-8

ISSN: 0065-3446

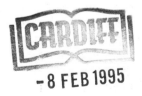
Printed in Great Britain by BPCC Wheatons Ltd, Exeter

PREFACE

In recent years, siginificant advances have been made in research in the field of the peripheral actions of dopamine, namely on its importance in the development and maintenance of some pathological conditions. As occurred in many other areas of scientific knowledge, a considerable part of which is known today on *peripheral dopamine* is the result of a stimulating exchange of ideas held on occasions where discussions between physiologists, pharmacologists, and clinicians were made possible. Previous editions of *"Dopamine Conferences"* have been successful in bringing together those interested in the peripheral actions of dopamine and it is our belief that in its 4th edition the main purpose of these kinds of meetings has been achieved. The present volume comprises the proceedings of the *"4th International Conference on Peripheral Dopamine"* held in Porto (Portugal), 18-20 June, 1992, and contains information on recent developments in the research on *peripheral dopamine*, particularly that concerning the renal and cardiovascular actions of the amine.

The first part of the book contains full reports on the following themes: sources, metabolism and fate of endogenous dopamine; dopamine receptors, their molecular biology and transduction pathways, localization and involvement in the control of sympathetic activity; dopamine, blood pressure and sodium homeostasis, and finally on the utilization of dopamine receptor agonists and dopamine prodrugs in cardiovascular and renal diseases. The second part of the book includes the abstracts of poster presentations which have addressed pertinent questions on the renal actions of dopamine, sodium homeostatis, sympathetic neurotransmission, dopamine, hypertension and diabetic nephropathy, and the pharmacodynamic and pharmacokinetic profile of new dopamine receptor agonists.

The *"Proceedings of the Dopamine Conference"* offer an up-to-date review of the current knowledge on the peripheral actions of dopamine, the role of renal dopamine in water and electrolyte

Advances in the Biosciences Vol. 88
© 1993 Pergamon Press Ltd.
Printed in Great Britain.

homeostasis, the relevance of peripheral dopaminergic mechanisms in the development and maintenance of some cardiovascular and renal disorders and confronts both basic scientists and clinicians with important questions which hopefully may be solved in the near future.

As the Editor of the present volume I would like to express my gratitude to Professor Walter Osswald for his most stimulating support, encouragement and guidance. Our effort in editing the present volume is dedicated to him, on the occasion of his retirement.

P. Soares-da-Silva
Porto, Portugal

ACKNOWLEDGEMENTS

This volume presents the proceedings of the "**4th International Conference on Peripheral Dopamine**" held in Porto, Portugal, in June 1992. This conference was organized with the financial support of Faculdade de Medicina do Porto, Faculdade de Medicina Dentária do Porto, Reitoria da Universidade do Porto, Instituto Nacional de Investigação Científica (INIC), Câmara Municipal do Porto, Fundação Luso-Americana para o Desenvolvimento, Fundação Calouste Gulbenkian, Commission of the European Communities, Laboratórios Bial, SmithKline Beecham Pharmaceuticals, Zambon Research, Inpharzam Nederland and Glaxo Farmacêutica, Lda (Portugal).

Contents

Contents

Involvement of Endogenous Dopamine in Control of Renal Function

C. Bell

Department of Physiology, University of Melbourne Medical Centre,
Parkville, Victoria 3052, Australia

ABSTRACT

Activation of specific dopamine receptors in the renal microvasculature and on tubular epithelial cells elevates effective renal plasma flow, glomerular filtration and urine formation and reduces sodium reabsorption. Data from rat and man also shows that dopamine is released within the kidney during renal compensation for salt and water loads. The effects of dopamine receptor antagonists and synthesis inhibitors support the view that endogenous dopamine is essential for the normal compensatory responses to salt and volume loads. In rat and dog, neural dopamine is likely to mediate the vascular actions while tubular synthesis is the primary natriuretic agent. In man, however, the balance between neural and non-neural mechanisms is less clear. While many details of the actions and origins of the endogenous dopamine are still to be resolved, there are likely to be important physiological and pathophysiological roles for this amine in controlling fluid balance.

INTRODUCTION

Over the last 10 years, a substantial body of data has accumulated to confirm the importance of DA as an intrarenal modulator of salt and water excretion, and to suggest the involvement of defects within the renal dopaminergic system in certain disorders of circulatory and renal control. The intense interest in this area has been reflected in the fact that, since 1986, five major international meetings in the area have been held.

Three main lines of evidence can be followed in the development of the theme of renal dopaminergic mechanisms - the identification of intrarenal DA

© 1993 Pergamon Press Ltd.
Printed in Great Britain.

C. Bell

receptors that mediate characteristic effects, the correlation of intrarenal DA
release with renal capacity for salt and water clearance and the demonstration that
inhibitors of DA production or action modify renal function. Molecular biology
continues to generate rapid advances in our knowledge of the DA receptors and, as
other articles in this volume provide the latest information on the topic, I will not
attempt to summarize it here. Rather, I shall attempt to summarize the current
status of DA as an intrarenal hormone and identify some possible avenues for
future productive investigation.

RENAL DA AND SODIUM EXCRETION

In the rat, it is now incontrovertible that natriuretic capacity following
moderate (2-5% body weight) iso-osmotic volume loading can be correlated with
urinary DA clearance [1-4]. The natriuretic response appears clearly to be
mediated by DA since treatment with DA antagonists, either of non-selective or
selective DA-1 types, or inhibition of dopa decarboxylation, reduce the ability to
excrete salt. The importance of DA in natriuresis may depend critically on the
degree of loading, as it has been shown that larger (10-20% body weight) volume
loads induce a natriuresis that is far less sensitive to inhibition of DA synthesis or
action and is associated with smaller or no increments in DA excretion [1,2].

In the Dahl and SHR strains of rat with hereditary predispositions to
hypertension, studies of the effects on blood pressure of renal transplantation
suggest an association of renal dysfunction with the development of hypertension
[see 5] and several groups have recently studied the renal DA system in these
strains. Reports of *in vitro* investigations suggest that defective coupling may exist
between the renal DA-1 receptor and its second messenger system in SHR [6-8].
However, *in vivo* inhibition of DA synthesis further elevates blood pressure in this
strain [7], suggesting that there may be tonic activation of the dopaminergic
system. As well, the natriuretic capacity of SHR kidneys when challenged with
sodium loads appears normal or even exaggerated [4]. On the other hand, urinary
DA excretion during salt loading may be defective in Dahl rats [7,9].

In slightly volume-expanded human subjects, both the selective DA-2
antagonist metoclopramide and the non-selective DA antagonist sulpiride reduce
sodium excretion without affecting renal plasma flow or glomerular filtration [10-
12]. The effect of sulpiride seems likely to have been mediated via DA-2 receptors

because there was no attenuation of renal vasodilator responses to exogenous DA [12]. The site of this antinatriuretic action is not clear. With metoclopramide, plasma aldosterone (PAC) was observed to rise [11], consistent with antagonism of the tonic dopaminergic inhibition of adrenocortical secretory activity that has been documented by other workers [13-15]. Aldosterone levels were not assessed following sulpiride, but the rise in potassium excretion seen was compatible with alteration of aldosterone secretion [12]. While the pharmacological data suggest that renal vascular receptors for DA in both man and dog are least predominantly of the DA-1 type [16], it is of interest that the selective DA-1 receptor antagonist SCH 23390 has been found, in conscious dogs, to produce natriuresis and diuresis without affecting renal plasma flow [17]. In the same model, a selective antagonist at DA-2 receptors was found to cause both elevated blood flow and enhanced salt and water excretion [18].

It is intriguing that a series of patients with mild renal failure were found to have higher PACs than control subjects and to not exhibit any further elevation of aldosterone with metoclopramide [11]. As well, a study of salt-resistant and salt-sensitive hypertensive patients found that PAC was increased by metoclopramide only in the salt-resistant population [19].

Recent studies continue to confirm earlier reports [20,21] that the capacity to excrete salt loads in man is correlated with renal production of DA and is proportional to urinary DA excretion [22,23]. Further, the observation of Harvey and colleagues [21] that some essential hypertensive patients exhibit an impaired ability to produce renal DA and to excrete salt, has also been repeatedly confirmed. One recent study [22] reported that these salt-sensitive patients show an enhanced capacity for urinary excretion of DOPA and suggested that this may reflect impaired renal capacity for uptake or conversion of DOPA at intrarenal sites. In normotensives with a family history of essential hypertension, a second recent study also concluded that there was likely to be defective renal conversion of plasma DOPA into DA [23]. This group of patients also exhibited subnormal resting urinary DA and an augmented natriuretic response to exogenous DA. A number of studies have previously noted that circulating DA and, more consistently, the ratio of plasma DA to noradrenaline (DA:NE) is decreased in essential hypertensives [see 24].

SOURCES OF RENAL DA

Comparisons of plasma amine concentrations in samples taken under circumstances in which large changes in circulating NE and adrenaline (EPI) occur show convincingly that the sympathetic vasoconstrictor nerves are not the primary source of plasma DA. For example, upright tilting is associated with rises in both NE and EPI of about two-fold, while DA is elevated by only about 20% [25-28]. Similarly, the profound rise in plasma NE seen in pheochromocytoma patients is not associated with comparable rises in circulating DA [29,30]. Overall, the plasma data available are closely in line with those based on more direct measurements in animal studies, and indicate that the ratio of DA:NE released from noradrenergic nerve endings is about 1:100 [31]. The situation with respect to adrenomedullary release is less clear, but it is unlikely that the ratio would be substantially different from that for sympathetic nerves.

Sampling from arterial and from central and peripheral venous sites indicates that a large proportion of plasma DA originates from organs located within the core of the body. Of these, the adrenal medulla seems an unlikely candidate, for the reasons discussed above, and little catecholamine efflux is thought to arise from the brain [32], so visceral organs are likely to contribute most of this DA, with the kidney a primary candidate. Even though the kidney cannot be the sole source of DA in the circulating pool [27], it is therefore likely that comparisons of peripheral and central venous DA levels provides an index of renal release.

The origin of the intrarenal DA remains a subject of some controversy. The large amounts of DA excreted into the urine, together with the demonstrable filtration of plasma DOPA into tubular fluid, the presence of tubular epithelial DOPA decarboxylase and the correlation of these processes with DA excretion, make a non-neural tubular source the likely predominant source of urinary DA in rat, dog and man [33-35]. Nevertheless, surgical denervation of rat kidney decreases urinary DA excretion by about one-third [36] and impairs the natriuretic response to salt load [37]. Ziegler and colleagues have demonstrated that, in chronically denervated (transplanted) human kidneys, DA is reduced by about two-thirds relative to those of control subjects, although NE excretion is similar in both groups [38]. Acute surgical denervation of dog kidneys results in virtual abolition of DA efflux into renal venous plasma [39], suggesting that tubular DA contributes minimally to this. In human subjects with denervated kidneys, Zeigler *et al.* [38]

found that plasma DA was only about 25% of that in control subjects, but this did not reach statistical significance because of an exceptionally high degree of variability in the control population.

In the rat, Baines & Drangova [40] found that renal denervation reduced glomerular filtration although, as this experiment involved isolated perfused kidneys, the data are difficult to interpret. In dog, selective electrical activation of the dopaminergic renal nerves elevates renal plasma flow and glomerular filtration, but does not cause natriuresis [41]. Neurally released DA also appears to participate in the renal vasodilation essential for autoregulation during reduced arterial perfusion pressure [42,43].

All these data are consistent with the view that neurogenic DA is involved primarily with regulation of renal perfusion and formation of filtrate, while regulation of tubular sodium reabsorption involves extraneuronal DA formed in the tubular wall. Such a division of responsibilities is compatible with the observed distribution of intrarenal dopaminergic nerve fibres, which predominantly supply vascular structures in the dog [44] and appear not to supply tubules at all in the rat [45]. It remains an open question however, how relevant this schema is to the situation in human kidney. The studies using DA receptor blockers suggest that endogenous DA participates in control of tubular function but not in control of GFR [10-12], despite the presence of vascular DA receptors [16] with effects similar to those sen in rat and dog. There is a similar difference in distribution of dopaminergic nerves which, by contrast with the cortical localization in rat and dog, are restricted to the medullary vasa recta in man [46]. Functionally, the dramatic effects of denervation on renal DA production [38] must be considered, as well as the apparent reflex release of DA from the kidney, independent of NE, during systemic cardiovascular adjustments in normal subjects [47]. Thus, although at present there are no data that overwhelmingly favour either neural or non-neural processes as the dominant dopaminergic pathway in human kidney, dopaminergic nerves must be considered likely to have some role.

SOME FUTURE DIRECTIONS

Practicalities predominate in any considerations of future studies. Despite the valuable information that it has provided, urinary DA must be regarded as an imprecise and unsatisfactory index of renal DA production, subject to distortion by diet and by other factors. It is therefore vital to refine the methodologies for measurement of plasma DA, so that it is no longer at the limits of resolution. In association with this, more thought should be given to simultaneous sampling from peripheral and central veins, in order to obtain indices that more accurately reflect DA of renal origin.

Clarifying the functional role of DA in man is necessarily difficult because of ethical constraints. Nevertheless, the initiative shown by Ziegler and colleagues [38] should serve as a stimulus for other workers to try to identify patient populations where, by virtue of disease or of surgical history, valid information on the mechanisms of intrarenal regulation might be obtained.

A host of other questions remain: is the DA-2-mediated natriuretic response renal or adrenal in location? Which of the intrarenal sites known to possess DA receptors are normally exposed to endogenous DA? Does DA participation in the human response to volume loading depend on the degree of expansion, as seems to occur in rat? If so, what mediates the DA-independent component? Are the sensors that initiate the dopaminergic response responding to sodium or to volume, and is this mechanism species-specific [see 32]? Are there any patient groups in whom DA is an essential component of renal regulation? If so, what implications does this have for their drug therapy? Are there groups, such as the aged [48-50] in whom loss of endogenous dopaminergic function has prejudiced renal control?

Perhaps later speakers at this meeting will already begin to answer some of these concerns: in any case, it is certain that these Proceedings will reinforce awareness of the potential importance of renal DA in a variety of clinical circumstances.

ACKNOWLEDGEMENTS

Work in my laboratory is currently supported by the National Health and Medical Research Council of Australia and the Helen M Schutt Trust.

REFERENCES

1. Chen, C.-J., Lokhandwala, M.F. Role of endogenous dopamine in the natriuretic response to various degrees of iso-osmotic volume expansion in rats, Clin. Exp. Hypert. 1991; A13: 1117-1126.

2. Bass, A.S., Murphy, M.B. Selective role of dopamine in the natriuresis produced by iso-osmotic saline infusion, Clin. Exp. Hypert. 1991; A13: 1127-1151.

3. Hegde, S.S., Jadhav, A.L., Lokhandwala, M.F.. Role of kidney dopamine in the natriuretic response to volume expansion in rats, Hypertension 1989; 13: 828-834.

4. Hansell, P., Sjöquist, M. Dopamine receptor blockade and synthesis inhibition during exaggerated natriuresis in spontaneously hypertensive rats, Acta Physiol. Scand. 1992; 144: 269-276.

5. De Wardener, H.E. The primary role of the kidney and salt intake in the aetiology of essential hypertension: part I, Clin. Sci. 1990; 79: 193-200.

6. Chen, C.-J., Vyas, S.J., Eichberg, J., Lokhandwala, M.F. Diminished phospholipase C activation by dopamine in spontaneously hypertensive rats, Hypertension 1992; 19: 102-108.

7. Yoshimura, M., Ikegaki, I., Nishimura, M., Takahashi, H. Role of dopaminergic mechanisms in the kidney for the pathogenesis of hypertension, J. Auton. Pharmac. 1990; 10, suppl. 1: s67-s72.

8. Kinoshita, S., Sidhu, A., Felder, R.A. Defective dopamine-1 receptor adenylate cyclase coupling in the proximal convoluted tubules from the spontaneously hypertensive rat, J. Clin. Invest. 1989; 84: 1849-1858.

9. De Feo, M.L., Jadhav, A.L., Lokhandwala, M.F., Dietary sodium intake and sodium excretion during the course of blood pressure development in Dahl salt-sensitive and salt-resistant rats, Clin. Exp. Hypert. 1987; A9: 2049-2060.

10. Krishna, G.G., Danovitch, G.M., Sowers, J.R. Catecholamine responses to central volume expansion produced by head-out water immersion and saline infusion, Clin. Endocrinol. Metab. 1983; 56: 998-1002.

11. Smit, A.J., Meijer, S., Wesseling, H., Donker, A.J.M., Reitsma, W.D. Effect of metoclopramide on dopamine-induced changes in renal function in healthy controls and in patients with renal disease, Clin. Sci. 1988; 75: 421-428.

12. Smit, A.J., Meijer, S., Wesseling, H., Donker, A.J.M., Reitsma, W.D. Disocciation of renal vasodilator and natriuretic effects of dopamine during sulpiride infusion in normal man, Eur. J. Clin. Pharmac. 1990; 39: 221-226.

13. Carey, R.M., Thorner, M.O., Ortt, E.M. Effects of metoclopramide and bromocriptine on the renin-angiotensin-aldosterone system in man, J. Clin. Invest. 1979; 63: 727-735.

14. Whitfield, L., Sowers, J.R., Tuck, M.L., Golub, M.S. Dopaminergic control of plasma catecholamine and aldosterone responses to acute stimuli in normal man, J. Clin. Endocrinol. Metab. 1980; 51: 724-729.

15. Lombardi, C., Missale, C., De Cotiis, R., Spedini, C., Pizzoccolo, G., Memo, M., Albertini. A., Spano, P.F. Inhibition of the aldosterone response to sodium depletion in man by stimulation of dopamine DA_2 receptors, Eur. J. Clin. Pharmac. 1988; 35: 323-326.

16. Kohli, J.D., Goldberg, L.I. The vascular (DA_1) dopamine receptor, in Peripheral Actions of Dopamine, Bell, C., McGrath, B. eds., Macmillan Press: London, 1988; pp. 108-123.

17. Siragy, H.M., Felder, R.A., Howell, N.L., Chevalier, R.L., Peach, M.J., Carey, R.M. Evidence that intrarenal dopamine acts as a paracrine substance at the renal tubule, Am. J. Physiol. 1989; 257: F469-F477.

18. Siragy, H.M., Felder, R.A., Howell, N.L., Chevalier, R.L., Peach, M.J., Carey, R.M. Evidence that dopamine-2 mechanisms control renal function, Am. J. Physiol. 1990; 259: F793-F800.

19. Shikuma, R., Yoshimura, M., Kambara, S., Yamazaki, H., Takashina, R., Takahashi, H., Takeda, K., Ijichi, H. Dopaminergic modulation of salt sensitivity in patients with essential hypertension, Life Sci. 1986; 38: 915-921.

20. Alexander, R.W., Gill, J.R. Jr., Yamabe, H., Lovenberg, W., Keiser, H.R. Effects of dietary sodium and of acute saline infusion on the interrelationship between dopamine excretion and adrenergic activity in man, J. Clin. Invest. 1974; 54: 194-200.

21. Harvey, J.N., Casson, I.F., Clayden, A.D., Cope, G.F., Perkins, C.M., Lee, M.R. A paradoxical fall in urine dopamine output when patients with essential hypertension are given added dietary salt, Clin. Sci. 1984; 67: 83-88.

22. Gill, J.R. Jr., Grossman, E., Goldstein, D.S. High urinary dopa and low urinary dopamine-to-dopa ratio in salt-sensitive hypertension, Hypertension 1991; 18: 614-621.

23. Iimura, O., Shimamoto, K., Suppressed dopaminergic activity and water-sodium handling in the kidneys at the prehypertensive stage of essential hypertension, J. Auton. Pharmac. 1990; 10, suppl. 1: s73-s77.

24. Bell, C. Peripheral dopaminergic nerves, in Novel Peripheral Neurotransmitters, Bell, C. ed., Pergamon Press: New York, 1991; pp. 135-160.

25. Kjeldson, S. E., Flaaten, B., Eide, I., Helgeland, A., Leren, P., Fonstelien, E., Decreased peripheral dopaminergic activity in essential hypertension? Scand. J. Clin. Lab. Invest. 1983; 43: 15-20.

26. Kjeldson, S.E., Flaaten, B., Eide, I., Helgeland, A., Leren, P. Evidence of increased peripheral catecholamine release in patients with long-standing, untreated essential hypertension, Scand. J. Lab. Invest. 1982; 42: 217-223.

27. Miura, Y., Takahashi, M., Sano, N., Ohzeki, T., Mefuro, Y., Sugawara, T., Noshiro, T., Watanabe, H., Shimizu, K., Abe, K., Yoshinaga, K. Plasma free dopamine in human hypertension, Clin. Exp. Hypert. 1989; A11, Suppl. 1: 227-236.

28. Hallbrügge, T., Gerhardt, T., Ludwig, J., Heidbreder, E., Graefe, K.-H. Assay of catecholamines and dihydroxyphenylethyleneglycol in human plasma and its application in orthostasis and mental stress, Life Sci. 1988; 43: 19-26.

29. Kuchel, O., Buu, N.T., Fontaine, A., Hamet, P., Beroniade, V., Larochelle, P., Genest, J. Free and conjugated plasma catecholamines in hypertensive patients with and without pheochromocytoma, Hypertension 1980; 2: 177-186.

30. Miura, Y., Takahashi, M., Sano, N., Kimura, S., Toriyabe, S., Ishizuka, Y., Noshiro, T., Ohashi, H., Sugawara, T., Watanabe, H., Yoshinaga, K., DeQuattro, V. Plasma levels of unconjugated dopamine in various types of hypertension, J. Cardiovasc. Pharmac. 1987; 10, suppl. 4: S167-S169.

31. Bell, C. Dopamine release from sympathetic nerve terminals, Prog. Neurobiol. 1988; 30: 193-208.

32. Bell, C. Endogenous renal dopamine and control of blood pressure, Clin. Exp. Hypert. 1987; A9: 955-976.

33. Baines, A.D., Chan, W. Production of urine free dopamine from dopa: a micropuncture study, Life Sci. 1980; 26: 253-259.

34. Brown, M.J., Allison, D.J. Renal conversion of plasma DOPA to urine dopamine, Br. J. Clin. Pharmac. 1981; 12: 251-253.

35. Zimlichman, R., Levinson, P.D., Kelly, G., Stull, R., Keiser, H.R., Goldstein, D.S. Derivation of urinary dopamine from plasma dihydroxyphenylalanine, Clin. Sci. 1988; 75: 515-520.

36. Stephenson, R.K., Sole, M.J., Baines, A.D., Neural and extraneural catecholamine production by rat kidney, Am. J. Physiol. 1982; 242: F261-F266.

37. Grossman, E., Hoffman, A., Chang, P.C., Keiser, H.R., Goldstein, D.S. Increased spillover of dopa into arterial blood during dietary salt loading, Clin. Sci. 1990; 78: 423-429.

38.   Ziegler, M.G., Morrissey, E.C., Kennedy, B., Elayen, H. Sources of urinary catecholamines in renal denervated transplant recipients, J. Hypert. 1990; 8: 927-932.

39.   Petrovic, T., Harris, P.J., Bell, C. Comparison of resting and stimulus-evoked catecholamine release from the femoral and renal vascular beds of the dog, J. Auton. Nerv. Syst. 1988; 25: 195-176.

40.   Baines, A.D., Drangova, R. Neural not tubular dopamine increases glomerular filtration rate in perfused rat kidney, Am. J. Physiol. 1986; 250: F674-F679.

41.   Bell, C., Sunn, N. A functional role for renal dopaminergic nerves in the dog, J. Auton. Pharmac. 1990; 10, suppl. 1: s41-s46.

42.   Kapusta, D.R., Robie, N.W. Plasma dopamine in regulation of canine renal blood flow, Am. J. Physiol. 1988; 255: R379-R387.

43.   Sunn, N., Woodman, O.L., Bell, C. Involvement of dopamine in control of renal blood flow, J. Auton. Nerv. Syst. 1992; in press.

44.   Ferguson, M., Ryan, G.B., Bell, C. The innervation of the dog renal cortex: an ultrastructural study, Cell Tissue Res. 1988; 253: 539-546.

45.   Ferguson, M., Bell, C. Two patterns of DOPA decarboxylase immunoreactivity in sympathetic axons supplying rat renal cortex, Renal Physiol. Biochem. 1991; 14: 55-62.

46.   Bell, C., Bhathal, P.S., Mann, R., Ryan, G.B. Evidence that dopaminergic sympathetic axons supply the medullary arterioles in human kidney, Histochemistry 1989; 91: 361-364.

47.   Tingren, B., Hjemdahl, P., Theodorsson, E., Nussberger, J. Renal responses to lower body negative pressure, Am. J. Physiol. 1990; 259: F573-F579.

48.   Kuchel, O. Peripheral dopamine in pathophysiology of hypertension: interaction with aging and lifestyle, Hypertension 1991; 18: 709-721.

49.   Ricci, A. The renal dopaminergic system in ageing, J. Auton. Pharmac. 1990; 10, suppl. 1: s19-s24.

50.   Fancourt, G.J., Asokan, V.,S., Bennett, S.C., Walls, J., Castleden, C.M. The effects of dopamine and a low protein diet on glomerular filtration rate and renal plasma flow in the aged kidney, Eur. J. Clin. Pharmac. 1992; 42: 375-378.

The Intestinal Mucosa as a Source of Dopamine

A.M. Bertorello*, M.A. Vieira-Coelho[†],
A.C. Eklöf*, Y. Finkel* and P. Soares-da-Silva[†]

*Department of Pediatrics, Karolinska Institutet, St Goran's
Children's Hospital, Stockholm, Sweden
[†]Department of Pharmacology and Therapeutics, Faculty of
Medicine, Porto, Portugal

ABSTRACT

The present work reports on the formation of dopamine along the rat digestive tract under *in vitro* experimental conditions and on the levels of endogenous dopamine and the turnover rate of the amine in the jejunal mucosa of developing rats. The basal levels of endogenous dopamine were similar in the non-glandular and glandular stomach, duodenum, jejunum and ileum; they were found to be higher in the proximal colon and lower in the distal colon. The synthesis of dopamine from added L-DOPA (500 µM) was found to be in the duodenum, jejunum and ileum 2-fold that in the proximal colon, 6-fold that in the glandular stomach and 120-fold that in the non-glandular stomach and the distal colon. The synthesis of dopamine in tissues loaded with exogenous L-DOPA was not accompained by an increased formation of noradrenaline. The basal levels of DOPA and dopamine in the jejunal mucosa were found in 20 day-old rats to be, respectively, 5- and 2-fold those observed in older animals. When challenged with a high sodium diet both 20 and 40 day-old rats were found to present higher levels of endogenous dopamine in the mucosa, but not of DOPA; the increase in dopamine levels observed during a HS diet was similar in 20 and in 40 day-old rats (respectively, 75% and 67% increase). During inhibition of AAAD with benserazide, the rate of DOPA accumulation in the jejunal mucosa was found to be similar in 20 day-old rats (k=0.040±0.004) and 40 day-old rats (k=0.042±0.004); the total amount of DOPA accumulated during AAAD inhibition was, however, considerably greater in 20 day-old rats (1324±156 pmol g^{-1}) than in 40 day-old rats (247±28 pmol g^{-1}).

INTRODUCTION

Increasing evidence over the past few years has suggested that dopamine, through the activation of specific receptors, may modulate a variety of functions of the digestive tract such as secretion of gastrointestinal fluids, absorption of electrolytes and fluids, motility and control of blood flow (for review see 1). The physiological relevance of these actions depends, however, on the location and on the amount and availability of the endogenous dopamine to activate the specific receptors for the amine. Some of dopamine in the gastrointestinal tract is used for the synthesis of noradrenaline, but most of the amine has been demonstrated to be insensitive to chemical and surgical denervation procedures (2,3,4); this would suggest that the amine may be stored in a non neuronal compartment. Moreover, in the sparsely innervated mucosa of the dog duodenum, jejunum and ileum the proportion of dopamine to noradrenaline was found to be twice that in the muscular layers and denervation by 6-hydroxydopamine produced a further increase in this ratio (2).

The formation of dopamine in non neuronal elements has been ascribed to chromaffin cells in a variety of tissues and organs; in renal tissues, however, most of dopamine located in non neuronal elements has been demonstrated to be synthetized in epithelial cells of proximal tubules (5,6). These cells are endowed with a high AAAD activity and synthetize dopamine from 3,4-dihydroxyphenylalanine (DOPA) present in the tubular filtrate; the amine thus formed has been shown to be of particular importance in the renal handling of water and electrolytes (7). The cellular uptake of L-DOPA occurs through an energy-dependent and stereoselective carrier-mediated process (8) and evidence produced subsequently favours the view that the synthesis of dopamine in tubular epithelial cells is in fact submitted to some sort of regulation. Firstly, it was described that sodium loading is accompanied by an increased excretion of dopamine in the urine of either humans and laboratory animals (9-12) and that a low sodium diet results in a decrease in the urinary excretion of dopamine (6,11,12). In line with this view, it has been recently reported in both human and rat kidney preparations that the production of dopamine is not only closely dependent on extracellular sodium, but also appears to be related to the transtubular reabsorption of sodium (13) and on the integrity of the tubular cytoskeleton and the functional integrity of the Na^+-K^+-ATPase (14).

The intestinal tract has also been shown to be of crucial importance in the regulation of body water and electrolyte homeostasis with particular relevance in the control of changes in fluid and electrolyte intake (15). The intestine, namely its duodenal and ileal portions, have been demonstrated to be endowed with a considerable AAAD activity (16,17), namely located in non neuronal cellular elements (16,18), and there is evidence to suggest that dopamine may be implicated in the regulation of water and electrolyte absorption in this organ (19). The present study reports on the formation of dopamine along the rat digestive tract under in vitro experimental conditions and on the levels of endogenous dopamine and the turnover rate of the amine in the jejunal mucosa of developing rats. In some experiments, rats were given a high sodium (HS) diet, a manoeuvre known to stimulate the formation of dopamine in epithelial cells of the renal proximal tubules (20).

MATERIALS and METHODS

Male Wistar rats (Biotério do Instituto Gulbenkian de Ciência, Oeiras, Portugal) aged 60 days and weighing 250-280 g or Sprague-Dawley rats (Anticimex, Sollentuna, Sweden), aged 20 and 40 days, weighing 50 to 150 g were used in the experiments. Animals were kept two to four per cage under controlled environmental conditions (12 h light/dark cycle and room temperature 24ºC). Food and tap water were allowed ad libitum. The experiments were all carried out during day time. The HS study group received 0.9% saline instead of tap water. The 20 day-old Sprague-Dawley rats on HS diet were fed for 4 days, while the 40 day-old animals received saline for 10 days prior to the study.

After anaesthesia the non-glandular and glandular stomach, duodenum, jejunum, ileum and proximal and distal colon were removed, open longitudinally with fine scissors and rinsed free from blood and the alimentary content with saline (0.9% NaCl). The selected tissues were placed on an ice-cold glass plate and fragments weighing 20 to 40 mg wet weight were prepared with fine scissors. Thereafter, the tissue fragments were preincubated for 30 min in 2 ml warm (37ºC) and gassed (95% O_2 and 5% CO_2) Krebs' solution. The Krebs' solution had the following composition (mM): NaCl 120, KCl 4.7, $CaCl_2$ 2.4, $MgSO_4$ 1.2, $NaHCO_3$ 25, KH_2PO_4 1.2, EDTA 0.4, ascorbic acid 0.57 and glucose 11; l-alpha-methyl-p-tyrosine (50 µM), tropolone (50 µM) and copper sulphate (10 µM) were also added to the Krebs' solution in order to inhibit the enzymes tyrosine hydroxylase and catechol-O-methyltransferase and to inhibit the endogenous inhibitors of dopamine ß-hydroxylase, respectively. After preincubation, tissues were incubated for 20 min in Krebs' solution with added L-DOPA (500 µM). The levels of dopamine and noradrenaline reflecting the control condition were determined in fragments of the selected tissues which have not been in contact with exogenous L-DOPA.

The basal levels of dopamine and the rate of utilization of endogenous DOPA was also determined in the jejunal mucosa of 20 and 40 day-old Sprague-Dawley rats. In some experiments, rats were tube-fed with benserazide (10 mg kg^{-1}), an inhibitor of AAAD, one hour before the sacrifice. After anaesthesia jejunal segments were removed, open longitudinally with fine scissors and rinsed free from blood and the alimentary content with saline (0.9% NaCl); the mucosa was gently removed with a salpel, placed in 0.5 ml 0.2 M perchloric acid and stored frozen until the assay of DOPA and dopamine. The accumulation of the precursor in the jejunal mucosa after inhibition of AAAD was calculated from a semilog plot of DOPA concentration against time of inhibition; the slope of accumulation was calculated using linear regression. The fractional rate constant of the accumulation of DOPA (k) was then obtained from the expression: k=slope value/0.434 (13).

The assay of L-DOPA, dopamine and noradrenaline was performed by means of high pressure liquid chromatography with electrochemical detection, as previously described (13). The lower limit for detection of noradrenaline, dopamine and DOPAC were, respectively, 750, 500 and 350 fmol 50 μl^{-1}.

RESULTS

As shown in table 1, the basal levels of noradrenaline were found to be similar in the non-glandular stomach, duodenum and jejunum and 30% lower in the glandular stomach, ileum and proximal and distal colon. The basal levels of endogenous dopamine were not significantly different in the non-glandular and glandular stomach, duodenum, jejunum and ileum; dopamine levels in the proximal colon were significantly higher than in all the other gastrointestinal areas studied, whereas the opposite was found for the distal colon. Incubation of non-glandular and glandular stomach, duodenum, jejunum, ileum and proximal and distal colon with exogenous L-DOPA (500 μM) during 20 min was found to result in a marked accumulation of newly-formed dopamine in the glandular stomach, duodenum, jejunum, ileum and proximal colon; in the non-glandular stomach and distal colon the production of dopamine from exogenous L-DOPA was found to be irrelevant in comparison with that observed in the duodenum, jejunum and ileum. The synthesis of dopamine was found to be in the duodenum, jejunum and ileum 2-fold that in the proximal colon, 6-fold that in the glandular stomach and 120-fold that in the non-glandular stomach and the distal colon. The synthesis of dopamine in tissues loaded with exogenous L-DOPA was in neither of the tissues analyzed accompanied by an increased formation of noradrenaline, in spite of the presence of 10 μM copper sulphate in the incubation medium.

As can be observed in figure 1a, the basal levels of DOPA and dopamine in the jejunal mucosa were found in 20 day-old rats to be, respectively, 5- and 2-fold those observed in older animals. When challenged with a HS diet both 20 and 40 day-old rats were found to present higher levels of endogenous dopamine in the mucosa; the increase in dopamine levels observed during a HS diet was similar in 20 (75% increase) and in 40 (67% increase) day-old rats. In both 20 and 40 day-old rats, the basal levels of DOPA in control animals were, however, similar to that found to occur in rats submitted to a HS diet. During inhibition of AAAD with benserazide (figure 1b), the rate constant of DOPA accumulation in the jejunal mucosa was found to be similar in 20 day-old rats (k=0.040±0.004) and 40 day-old rats (k=0.042±0.004); the total

Table 1. Levels of dopamine and noradrenaline (in nmol g^{-1}) in various gastrointestinal areas before and after incubation with L-DOPA (500 μM).

Tissue	DA Control	DA L-DOPA (500 μM)	NA Control	NA L-DOPA (500 μM)
Non-glandular stomach	0.18±0.02	2.0±0.6*	2.7±0.3	3.2±0.2
Glandular stomach	0.12±0.01	30.3±4.6*	1.9±0.2	2.4±0.2
Duodenum	0.17±0.02	176.0±38.4*	3.2±0.1	4.5±0.5
Jejunum	0.17±0.01	201.5±24.4*	3.0±0.3	5.2±0.6
Ileum	0.15±0.02	210.6±15.2*	1.8±0.2	5.4±0.4
Proximal colon	0.37±0.07#	102.8±18.8*	2.2±0.1	4.3±0.4
Distal colon	0.08±0.02#	1.65±0.7*	2.3±0.1	3.4±0.4

\# significantly different from corresponding values in the jejunum (P<0.02).

* significantly different from corresponding values in the absence of L-DOPA (P<0.01).

Figure 1. In (**A**) are shown the levels of endogenous 3,4-dihydroxyphenylalanine (DOPA; open columns) and dopamine (hatched columns) in 20 (n=12) and 40 (n=16) day-old rats. Some animals (n=5) were fed a normal salt diet and others (n=8) were fed a high salt diet (0.9 % saline in the drinking water). Each column represents the mean of 5-8 animals per group; vertical lines indicate S.E.M. values. Significantly different from corresponding values for NS rats (✱ P<0.01) and for corresponding values in 20 day-old rats (☆P<0.01). In (**B**) are shown the levels of DOPA in the jejunal mucosa of 20 (closed circles) and 40 (open circles) day-old rats at time 0 min and 60 min after the administration of 10 mg kg^{-1} benserazide. Results are shown for observations of the accumulation of DOPA; each point represents the mean of 8 animals per group; S.E.M. values were less than 10% of the correspoding means. Linear coefficient values were as follows: 20 day-old rats, r=0.996, n=16; 40 day-old rats, r=0.986, n=16.

A)

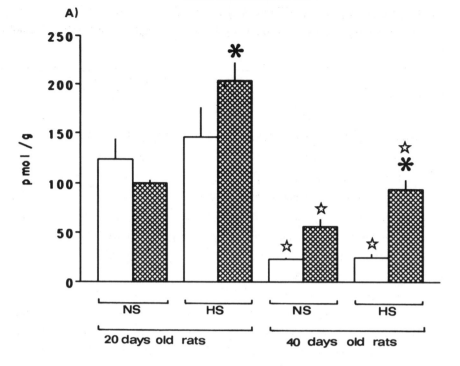

B)

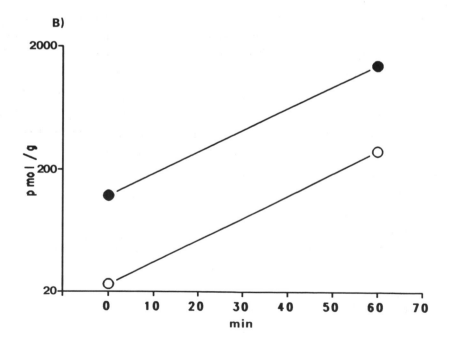

amount of DOPA accumulated during AAAD inhibition was, however, considerably greater in 20 day-old rats (1324 ± 156 pmol g^{-1}) than in 40 day-old rats (247 ± 28 pmol g^{-1}).

DISCUSSION

The present study shows that the ability to synthetize dopamine from exogenous L-DOPA is not the same along the rat digestive tract; the highest AAAD activity is located in the duodenum, jejunum, ileum, proximal colon and glandular stomach and is almost absent in the non-glandular and glandular stomach and distal colon. The increased levels of endogenous dopamine in the jejunal mucosa of 20 day-old rats appears to be the result of a high rate of decarboxylation of DOPA and the high delivery of sodium constitutes an important stimulus for the production of the amine in this area of the rat digestive tract.

The results reported here agree well with earlier evidence showing that the intestinal wall is of major importance in the first-pass metabolism of L-DOPA (16,17,18). Landsberg and Taubin (16) have also studied the uptake and metabolism of L-DOPA in several rat tissues including the digestive tract and found the duodenum and ileum of considerable importance in the decarboxylation of the dopamine precursor. These authors have stressed the need to clarify which type of cellular elements were responsible for the decarboxylation of L-DOPA and based on evidence obtained while employing 6-hydroxydopamine and reserpine did suggest that sympatetic nerves are not involved in the formation of dopamine from L-DOPA. The results obtained in the present study agree with the suggestion that sympathetic nerves do not represent an important alternative for the decarboxylation of L-DOPA; the main argument supporting this assumption is that no significant formation of noradrenaline was found to occur in parallel with the increase in the levels of dopamine, its imediate precursor. It should be stressed that the experimental conditions used would favour the hydroxylation of dopamine into noradrenaline; in fact, the reason to add 10 µM of copper sulphate was related to prevention of inhibition of dopamine ß-hydroxylase by the endogenous inhibitors of the enzyme (21). On the other hand, the finding that no significant formation of noradrenaline did occur from newly-formed dopamine with origin in exogenous L-DOPA supports the suggestion that decarboxylation does in fact take place mainly outside sympathetic nerves. Another result favouring the view that a considerable amount of the dopamine in the inestinal mucosa is non-neuronal in location is that denervation by 6-hydroxydopamine increases the proportion of dopamine to noradrenaline (2,3,4).

Although the present study produces no direct evidence of the type of cell responsible for the formation of dopamine from DOPA in the intestinal mucosa, it is, however, open to speculation the possibility that the cells responsible for the synthesis of dopamine are those of the intestinal epithelium, similarly to that occurring in the kidney. In fact, epithelial cells of the renal proximal convoluted tubules are, in contrast with those in the renal medulla, endowed with a high AAAD activity (6,22,23) and have been demonstrated to be the main source of dopamine production from filtered DOPA. The dopamine with origin in renal tubular epithelial cells has been suggested to be involved in the regulation of sodium tubular reabsorption (20,24-26); other types of evidence show, on the other hand, that sodium may as well be an important stimulus for the production of the amine (13,14). The results presented here on the jejunal mucosa agree with this view and show that the levels of endogenous dopamine in the jejunal mucosa were significantly increased in both 20 and 40 day-old rats after a short period of HS intake. This is in line with evidence presented for renal tissues by several authors, both under *in vitro* and *in vitro* experimental conditions (6,9-12,20,22). The fact that levels of DOPA in the jejunal mucosa of control rats were not different from those of animals fed a HS diet suggests that the mechanism(s) responsible for the increased production of dopamine is not related to an enhanced availability of the precursor. This would agree with that found to occur in renal tissues; the increased renal production of dopamine in animals given a HS diet has been demonstrated to be related to an increased activity of AAAD (6,22). An interesting finding, however, is that the percent increase of dopamine levels during HS intake was found to be similar in 20 and 40 day-old rats, though the levels of the amine in the jejunal mucosa of 20 day-old rats fed a NS diet were found to be twice those of 40 day-old animals. This difference does not appears to be related to differences in AAAD activity, since the rate constant of DOPA accumulation after inhibition of AAAD with benserazide was found to be similar in 20 (k=0.040±0.004) and in 40 day-old rats (k=0.042±0.004). Differences in the total amount of DOPA accumulated after benserazide indicate, on the other hand, a higher number of functional units decarboxylating DOPA into dopamine in 20 days in comparison with that occurring in 40 day-old rats. This would also explain why levels of endogenous dopamine levels in 20 day-old rats are greater than in older animals.

CONCLUSION

In conclusion, the results presented here demonstrate the presence of an heterogeneous pattern in the formation of dopamine along the digestive tract of the rat; the highest AAAD activities appear to be located in the duodenum, jejunum, ileum, proximal colon and glandular stomach and to be substantially lower in the non-glandular stomach and distal colon.   In the jejunal mucosa, the formation of dopamine is dependent on the dietary sodium and 20 day-old rats appear to have an increased number of dopamine synthetising units in comparison with older animals.

REFERENCES

1 - Lefebvre, R.A. Gastrointestinal dopamine receptors. In: Peripheral actions of dopamine. Bell C. & McGrath B. Macmillan Press, London, pp. 141-152, 1988.

2 - Esplugues, J.V., Caramona, M.M., Moura D. & Soares-da-Silva, P. Effects of chemical sympathectomy on dopamine and noradrenaline content of the dog gastrointestinal tract. J. Auton. Pharmacol. 1985;5:189-195.

3 - Graffner, H., Eklund, M., Hakanson, R. & Rosenberg, E. Effect of different denervation procedures on catecholamines in the gut. Scand. J. Gastroenterol. 1985;20:1276-1280.

4 - Eaker, E.Y., Bixler, G.B., Dunn, A.J., Moreshead, W.W. & Mathias, J.R. Dopamine and norepinephrine in the gastrointestinal tract of mice and the effects of neurotoxins.   J. Pharmacol. Exp. Ther. 1988;244:438-442.

5 - Baines, A.D. & Chan, W. Production of urine free dopamine from dopa: a micropuncture study. Life Sci. 1980;26:253-259.

6 - Hayashi, M., Yamaji, Y., Kitajima, W. & Saruta, T.   Aromatic L-amino acid decarboxylase activity along the rat nephron. Am. J. Physiol. 1990;258:F28-F33.

7 - Jose, P.A., Raymond, J.R., Bates, M.D., Aperia, A., Felder, R.A. & Carey, R.M. The renal dopamine receptors. J. Am. Soc. Nephrol. 1992;2:1265-1278.

8 - Chan, Y.L. Cellular mechanisms of renal tubular transport of L-DOPA and its derivatives in the rat: microperfusions studies. J. Pharmacol. Exp. Ther. 1974;199:17-24.

9 - Alexander, R.W., Gill, J.R. jr, Yamabe, H., Lovenberg, W. & Keiser, H.R. Effects of dietary sodium and acute saline infusion on the interelationship between dopamine excretion and adrenergic activity in man. J. Clin. Invest. 1974;54:194-200.

10 - Ball, S.G., Oates, N.S. & Lee, M.R. Urinary dopamine in man and rat: effects of inorganic salts on dopamine excretion. Clin. Sci. Mol. Med. 1978;55:167-173.

11 - Baines, A.D. Effects of salt intake and renal denervation on catecholamine catabolism and excretion. Kidney Int. 1982;21:316-322.

12 - Goldstein, D.S., Stull, R., Eisenhofer, G. & Gill, J.R. jr.   Urinary excretion of dihydroxyphenylalanine and dopamine during alterations of dietary salt intake in humans. Clin. Sci. 1989;76:517-522.

13 - Soares-da-Silva, P. & Fernandes, M.H. Sodium-dependence and ouabain-sensitivity of the synthesis of dopamine in renal tissues of the rat. Br. J. Pharmacol. 1992;105:811-816.

A.M. Bertorello et al.

14 - Soares-da-Silva, P.   Actin cytoskeleton, tubular sodium and the renal synthesis of dopamine. Biochem. Pharmacol. 1992;44:1883-1886.

15 - Binder, H.J.   Absorption and secretion of water and electrolytes by small and large intestine.   In: Gastrointestinal Disease (Sleisinger & Fordtran, Eds.) W.B. Saunders, Philadelphia, pp. 812-829, 1983.

16 - Landsberg, L. & Taubin, H.L.   Uptake and metabolism of L-3,4-dihydroxyphenylalanine (DOPA) in rat tissues. Biochem. Pharmacol. 1973;22:2789-2800.

17 - Iwamoto, K., Watanabe, J., Yamada, M., Atsumi, F. & Matsushita, T.   Effect of age on gastrointestinal and hepatic first-pass effects of levodopa in rats.   J. Pharm. Pharmacol. 1987;39:421-425.

18 - Soares-da-Silva, P.   Preferential decarboxylation of L-threo-3,4-dihydroxyphenylserine in rat renal tissues. Gen. Pharmacol. "in press".

19 - Donowitz M., Cusolito, S., Battisti, B., Fogel, R. & Sharp, G.W.   Dopamine stimulation of active Na and Cl absorption in rabbit ileum. J. Clin. Invest. 1982;69:1008-1016.

20 - Bertorello, A., Hokfelt, T., Goldstein, M. & Aperia, A.   Proximal tubule Na^+-K^+-ATPase activity is inhibited during high-salt diet: evidence for DA-mediated effect. Am. J. Physiol. 1988;254:F795-F801.

21 - Nelson D.L. & Molinoff, P.B.   Differential effects of nerve implulses on adrenergic nerve vesicles in rat heart. J. Pharmacol. Exp. Ther. 1976;198:112-122.

22 - Seri, I., Kone, B.C., Gullans, S.R., Aperia, A., Brenner, B.A. & Ballermann, B.J. Influence of Na^+ intake on dopamine-induced inhibition of renal cortical Na^+-K^+-ATPase. Am. J. Physiol. 1990;258:F52-F60.

23 - Soares-da-Silva, P. & Fernandes, M.H. Regulation of dopamine synthesis in the rat.   J. Auton. Pharmacol. 1990;10 (Suppl 1):s25-s30.

24 - Bertorello, A. & Aperia, A.   Short-term regulation of Na^+-K^+-ATPase activity by dopamine. Am. J. Hypertens. 1990;3:51S-54S.

25 - Bertorello, A. & Aperia, A.   Inhibition of proximal tubule Na^+-K^+-ATPase activity requires simultaneous activation of DA1 and DA2 receptors. Am. J. Physiol. 1990;259:F924-F928.

26 - Bertorello, A. & Aperia, A. Na^+-K^+-ATPase is an effector protein for protein kinase C in renal proximal tubule cells. Am. J. Physiol. 1989;256:F370-F373.

Sequential Involvement of Monoamine Oxidase and Catechol-O-Methyltransferase in the Metabolism of Newly-formed Dopamine in Rat Renal Tissues[1]

M. Helena Fernandes[2] and P. Soares-da-Silva

Department of Pharmacology and Therapeutics, Faculty of
Medicine, 4200 Porto, Portugal

ABSTRACT

The present study has examined the role of monoamine oxidase (MAO) and catechol-O-methyltransferase (COMT) in the metabolism of newly-formed dopamine. Rat renal cortical slices were incubated with L-3,4-dihydroxyphenylalanine (L-DOPA, 10 to 100 μM) for 15 min. Levels of dopamine and its deaminated (3,4-dihydroxyphenylacetic acid, DOPAC), methylated (3-methoxytyramine, 3-MT) and methylated plus deaminated (homovanillic acid, HVA; 3-methoxy-4-phenylethanol, MOPET) metabolites were determined by h.p.l.c. with electrochemical detection. A concentration dependent formation of dopamine and of its metabolites was observed. DOPAC was the major metabolite and lower levels of the methylated metabolites were obtained. Pargyline (100 μM) resulted in a 90% reduction in the formation of both DOPAC and HVA and in a 30% increase in the 3-MT/dopamine ratio; the total amount of metabolites formed was lower than in control conditions. These results suggest that deamination is more important than methylation in the metabolism of renal dopamine. However, methylation becomes quantitatively important when MAO is inhibited.

INTRODUCTION

In recent years, evidence suggesting that dopamine plays an important role in renal tissues, in the handling of water and electrolytes has been presented (1). Most of the dopamine formed in the kidney has its origin in non neuronal structures and results from the decarboxylation of filtered L-3,4-dihydroxyphenylalanine (L-DOPA) in tubular epithelial cells (2, 3). This is a quantitatively important process as tubular epithelial cells, namely those of the proximal convoluted tubules have a high aromatic amino acid decarboxylase (AAAD) activity (4, 5) and plasma levels of L-DOPA can attain concentrations up to 15 pmol ml-1 (6). The kidney, however, has one of the highest monoamine oxidase (MAO) activity in the body and the enzyme has been shown of importance in the metabolism of filtered monoamines (7, 8). MAO catalyses the oxidative deamination of catechol- and indolamines in mammalian tissues. The

© 1993 Pergamon Press Ltd.
Printed in Great Britain.

enzyme exists in two forms, MAO-A and MAO-B, which have been identified by their sensitivity to selective inhibitors and specific substrates (9). Catechol-O-methyltransferase (COMT), another key enzyme in the metabolism of monoamines, methylates a range of catechol derivatives including the catecholamines and their deaminated metabolites (10).

The metabolism of renal dopamine is a matter of particular importance because of the diuretic and natriuretic effects of the amine and inhibition of the renal catabolism of the amine is expected to potentiate its renal effects. Previous studies performed both under *in vitro* and *in vivo* experimental conditions have shown that MAO plays an important role in the metabolism of renal dopamine (11-13). In the human, rat and dog kidney, dopamine formed from L-DOPA, both in renal cortical slices and homogenates, is extensively metabolized to 3,4-dihydroxyphenylacetic acid (DOPAC), the deaminated derivative of dopamine. Also, high tissue levels of DOPAC were found in the cortex, outer medulla and inner medulla of rats given L-DOPA (13). In addition, studies in the rat kidney employing selective MAO-A and MAO-B inhibitors have demonstrated that both types of MAO are implicated in the deamination of renal dopamine, though it appeared that most of newly-formed dopamine is deaminated by MAO-A (11). Previous work on the specific activity of MAO-A and MAO-B in the cortex and the medulla of the human and rat kidney, as determined by radiochemical methods and using specific substrates, has shown that MAO-A is the predominant form of the enzyme in the rat kidney, whereas in the human kidney MAO-B activity closelly follows that of MAO-A (14).

The aim of the present work is to study the role of MAO and COMT in the metabolism of newly-formed dopamine in the rat kidney under *in vivo* and *in vitro* experimental conditions. For this purpose, the formation of dopamine and of its deaminated, methylated and deaminated plus methylated metabolites was determined in renal tissues of rats given L-DOPA and in renal cortical slices loaded with L-DOPA. The influence of MAO and COMT inhibitors in the metabolism of dopamine formed in these experimental conditions was also studied.

MATERIALS and METHODS

The formation of 3-O-methylDOPA (3-OMDOPA), dopamine, DOPAC, 3-methoxytyramine (3-MT), homovanillic acid (HVA) and 3-methoxyphenylethanol (MOPET) was studied in male Wistar rats (Biotério do Instituto Gulbenkian de Ciência, Oeiras, Portugal), 45-60 days old and weighing 200-280 g, given L-DOPA (30 mg kg[-1], i.p.) 15 min before sacrifice; the levels of these compounds were determined in three different areas of the kidney, the cortex and the outer and inner medulla. Sacrifice was performed under ether anaesthesia by decapitation and the kidneys removed after laparectomy through a midle line incision of the abdominal wall. Thereafter, the kidneys were rinsed in cold saline (0.9%) and fragments of the renal cortex and inner and outer medulla were dissected free with fine scissors. After dissection of the selected renal areas, tissues were placed in 2ml of 0.2M perchloric acid until quantification of dopamine and its metabolites.

The *in vitro* studies were performed in slices of rat renal cortex; animals were sacrificed by decapitation under ether anaesthesia and both kidneys removed and rinsed free from blood with saline. The kidneys were placed on an ice cold glass plate, the kidney poles removed and slices of renal cortex approximately 0.5 mm thick and weighing about 30 mg wet weight were prepared with a scalpel. Thereafter, renal slices were preincubated for 30 min in 2 ml warmed (37ºC) and gassed (95% O_2 and 5% CO_2) Krebs' solution. The Krebs' solution had the following composition (mM): NaCl 120, KCl 4.7, $CaCl_2$ 2.4, $MgSO_4$ 1.2, $NaHCO_3$ 25, KH_2PO_4 1.2, EDTA 0.4, ascorbic acid 0.57, glucose 10 and sodium butyrate 1; l-alpha-methyl-p-tyrosine (50 µM) and copper sulphate (10 µM) were also added to the Krebs' solution in order to inhibit the enzyme tyrosine hydroxylase and the endogenous inhibitors of dopamine ß-hydroxylase, respectively. After preincubation, renal slices were incubated for 15 min in Krebs' solution with increasing concentrations of L-DOPA (10 to 100 µM). The preincubation and incubation were carried out in glass test tubes, continuously shaken throughout the experiment. At the end of the incubation, the reaction was stopped by the addition of 250 µl 2 M perchloric acid and samples stored at 4ºC until the quantification of catecholamines, within the next 24 hours. In studies of MAO and COMT inhibition, renal cortical slices were incubated with 50 µM L-DOPA and the inhibitors, respectively pargyline (100 µM) and Ro 40-7592 (1 µM), were present during the preincubation and incubation periods.

The assay of L-DOPA, 3-OMDOPA, dopamine, DOPAC, 3-MT and HVA was performed by means of h.p.l.c. with electrochemical detection, as previously described (15).

Mean values ± s.e.mean of n experiments are given. Differences between two means were estimated by Students "t" test for unpaired data; a P value less than 0.05 was assumed to denote a significant difference.

RESULTS

The administration of L-DOPA 15 min before sacrifice results in a marked accumulation of newly-formed dopamine in all three renal areas under study. The tissue levels (in nmol g-¹) of dopamine in the renal cortex and the outer and inner medulla of rats given 30 mg kg-¹ of L-DOPA were, respectively, 157.9±20.4, 189.7±23.2 and 287.4±20.5. Expressing the results in nmoles of dopamine per gr of tissue it became apparent that a greater accumulation of the amine occurs in the inner medulla. However, since the medullary zone of the kidney does not express AAAD activity (3-5), this result may simply reflect the urinary excretion of dopamine formed in the proximal segments of the nephron. The major metabolite found to occur in the three renal areas was DOPAC, followed by HVA, 3-MT and MOPET. The levels of 3-OMDOPA were, in all three renal areas, very low; these were lower than those of L-DOPA, which reflect the amount of the substrate which was neither decarboxylated into dopamine nor methylated to 3-OMDOPA. In none of the three renal areas was the algebraic sum of the levels of methylated and methylated plus deaminated metabolites of dopamine (3-MT, HVA and MOPET) higher than the levels of DOPAC (figure 1A.).

Incubation of slices of renal cortex in the presence of increasing concentrations of L-DOPA resulted in a concentration-dependent formation of dopamine (figure 1B). The formation of dopamine metabolites, in these experimental conditions, was also found to be dependent on the concentration of L-DOPA present in the incubation medium; this, however, did not strictly parallel the formation of their parent amine, dopamine. The major metabolite of dopamine found to occur in these experimental conditions was DOPAC. In contrast with that reported under *in vivo* conditions, the levels of HVA were found to be less than half of those found for 3-MT in kidney slices loaded with L-DOPA. MOPET was not found detectable in these experimental conditions, even when the concentration of L-DOPA in the incubation medium was raised up to 100 μM.

Figure 2A shows results for the effect of pargyline (100 μM) and Ro 40-7592 (1.0 μM) on the formation of dopamine and its metabolites in renal cortical slices incubated with 50 μM L-DOPA for 15 min. Pargyline produced a 90% reduction in the formation of DOPAC and HVA; this effect was accompanied by an increase in the formation of dopamine (50% increase) and 3-MT (100% increase). A 30% increase in the 3-MT/dopamine ratio was also found to occur in conditions of MAO inhibition; values of the 3-MT/dopamine ratios were in control conditions and during MAO inhibition, respectively, 0.08±0.01 and 0.11±0.01. Inhibition of COMT with Ro 40-7592 in kidney slices loaded with 50 μM L-DOPA resulted in a decrease in the formation of the methylated metabolites (3-MT and HVA) (85% reduction) and in an increase in the formation of both DOPAC (62% increase) and dopamine (30% increase). The proportion of the total amount of amine metabolites (DOPAC+3-MT+HVA) to dopamine in kidney slices incubated with 50 μM L-DOPA was in the

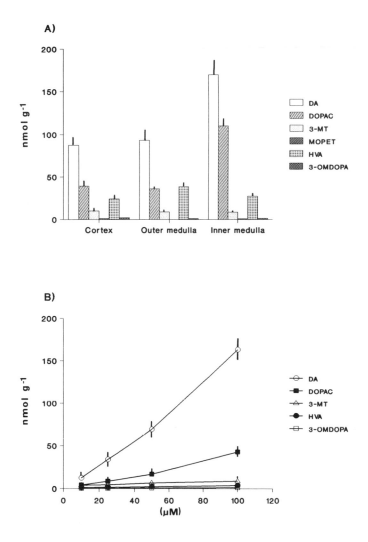

Figure 1. Levels (in nmol g⁻¹) of dopamine (DA), 3,4-dihydroxyphenylacetic acid (DOPAC), 3-methoxytyramine (3-MT), 3-methoxyphenylethanol (MOPET), homovanillic acid (HVA) and 3-O-methylDOPA (3-OMDOPA) in (**A**) the renal cortex, the outer and inner medulla of rats given L-DOPA (30 mg kg⁻¹, i.p.) 15 min before sacrifice and in (**B**) kidney slices incubated with increasing concentrations of L-DOPA (10 to 100 μM) for 15 min. Each column or each point represents the mean of five to seven experiments per goup; vertical lines show S.E.M..

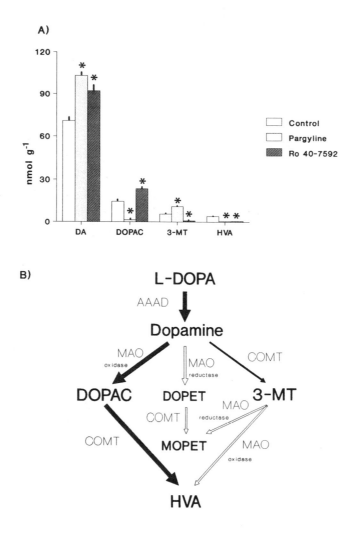

Figure 2. Part **A** shows the effect of pargyline (100 µM) and Ro 40-7592 (1 µM) on the accumulation of dopamine, 3,4-dihydroxyphenylacetic acid (DOPAC), 3-methoxytyramine (3-MT) and homovanillic acid (HVA) in slices of rat renal cortex loaded with 50 µM L-DOPA. Each column represents the mean of eight experiments per goup; vertical lines show S.E.M.. Significantly different from corresponding control values (* P<0.01). Part **B** is a schematic representation of the proposed metabolic pathway of newly-formed dopamine in rat renal tissues.

presence of pargyline (0.13±0.01) significantly lower (P<0.01) than that in controls (0.32±0.02) and in the presence of Ro 40-7592 (0.29±0.04).

DISCUSSION

Renal tissues are endowed with a considerable capacity to synthetize dopamine from L-DOPA, in both *in vivo* and *in vitro* experimental conditions. The newly-formed amine undergoes rapid metabolization by both MAO and COMT; however, deamination appears to be the main process involved in the degradation of the amine. In fact, the levels of DOPAC, in both *in vivo* and *in vitro* experimental conditions, were found to be significantly higher than the levels of the methylated and deaminated plus methylated metabolites. This suggests that in the kidney the relative importance of MAO in the metabolism of dopamine is greater than that of COMT, which contrasts with that described in vascular and other non-vascular tissues (16). Studies performed under *in vitro* experimental conditions on the formation of dopamine in three different species (human, dog and rat) have shown that renal tisssues have an enormous capacity to synthetize dopamine from L-DOPA and a significant amount of the newly-formed dopamine is deaminated to DOPAC (unplubished observations). The reduced role of COMT in the kidney is also reflected in the low levels of 3-OMDOPA formed from L-DOPA both under *in vivo* and *in vitro* experimental conditions, in comparison with the levels of dopamine, the product of the action of AAAD upon L-DOPA.

Since, almost all AAAD activity in the kidney is concentrated in the cortical area (4, 5, 17), namely in proximal convoluted tubules, it is expected that the formation of dopamine would be confined to the renal cortex. The levels of dopamine and of its metabolites were, however, in the outer and inner medulla even higher than those in the renal cortex; a possible explanation for this finding may be related to the presence of a high number of renal tubules per g of tissue in the medullary zones. Another interesting finding is that the proportion of dopamine to its metabolites in all three renal areas studied is very similar; considering that almost all of the dopamine present in the outer and inner medulla was synthetized in the cortex, this would favour the suggestion that no additional metabolism of dopamine has occurred from the momment the amine has been secreted into the tubular lumen. This may also agree with the view that the dopamine present in the tubular filtrate is not transported backwards into the tubular epithelial cell, as demonstrated by Chan (18).

The results obtained on the formation and metabolism of dopamine in the presence of pargyline also support the view that MAO plays an important role in the metabolism of newly-formed dopamine. Inhibition of MAO also resulted in a significant reduction in the formation of HVA; the magnitude of this effect was found to be similar to that for DOPAC. This is an expected result, since the formation of HVA, either through the methylation of DOPAC or the deamination of 3-MT, involves the enzyme MAO, which is particularly sensitive to pargyline. The relative importance of each pathway in the formation of HVA can not be deduced from the results obtained in the present study. However, they suggest that methylation of DOPAC into HVA is probably more important than the deamination of 3-MT into HVA. Two sets of results appear to support this suggestion: (1) the levels of DOPAC are higher than those of HVA and 3-MT; (2) in conditions of MAO inhibition, the reduction in the formation of DOPAC and HVA (corresponding to the loss of about 17 nmol g^{-1}) was not compensated by the increase in the formation of 3-MT (corresponding to an increase of about 5 nmol g^{-1}). However, the finding that in the presence of pargyline the proportion of 3-MT to dopamine increased by 30% agrees well with the view that, in conditions of MAO inhibition, methylation may become a quantitatively important process. In agreement with this suggestion is the finding that inhibition of COMT activity with Ro 40-7592 results in an increased accumulation of both dopamine and DOPAC in renal tissues loaded with L-DOPA. The metabolic pathway leading to the formation of MOPET appears to be endowed of minor importance, as the levels of this metabolite are very low or not detectable.

CONCLUSION

Renal dopamine is extensively metabolized by MAO and COMT as evidenced by the formation of deaminated and methylated metabolites of the amine. Deamination, however, appears to be more important than methylation and the predominant metabolic pathway of renal dopamine is most probably the deamination to DOPAC followed by its methylation to HVA (figure 2B). The results presented here suggest that inhibition of an important metabolic pathway in the degradation of renal dopamine may result in a potentiation of the diuretic and natriuretic effects of the amine.

REFERENCES

1 - Lee, M.R. Dopamine and the kidney. Clin. Sci. 1982;62:439-448.

2 - Baines, A.D. & Chan, W. Production of urine free dopamine from dopa: a micropuncture study. Life Sci. 1980;26:253-259.

3 - Suzuki, H.R., Nakane, H., Kawamura, M., Yoshizawa, M., Takeshita, E. & Saruta, T. Excretion and metabolism of dopa and dopamine by isolated perfused rat kideny. Am. J. Physiol. 1984;247:E285-E290.

4 - Hayashi, M., Yamaji, Y., Kitajima, W. & Saruta, T. Aromatic L-amino acid decarboxylase activity along the rat nephron. Am. J. Physiol. 1990;258:F28-F33.

5 - Seri, I., Kone, B.C., Gullans, S.R., Aperia, A., Brenner, B.M. & Ballermann, B.J. Influence of Na+ intake on dopamine-induced inhibition of renal cortical Na+-K+-ATPase. Am. J. Physiol. 1990;258:F52-F60.

6 - Cuche, J.L. Sources of circulating dopamine: a personal view. In peripheral actions of dopamine, ed. by Bell, C. & McGrath, B.P. pp. 1-23. London, Macmillan Press,1988.

7 - Stöcker, W. & Hempel , K. Inactivation and excretion of dopamine by the cat kidney in vitro. Naunyn-Schmiedeberg's Arch. Pharmacol. 1976;295:123-126.

8 - Kopin, I.J. Catecholamine metabolism: basic aspects and clinical significance. Pharmacol. Rev. 1985;37:333-364.

9- Youdim, M.B.H., Finberg, J.P.M. & Tipton, K.F. Monoamine oxidase. In Catecholamines, ed. by Trendelenburg, U. & Weiner, N., Vol. 1, pp.119-192, Springer-Verlag, Berlin, 1988.

10 - Nic a' Bháird, N., Goldberg, R. & Tipton, K.F. Catechol-O-methyltransferase and its role in metabolism. Adv. Neurol 1990;53:489-495.

11 - Fernandes, M.H. & Soares-da-Silva, P. Effects of MAO-A and MAO-B selective inhibitors Ro 41-1049 and Ro 19-6327 on the deamination of newly-formed dopamine in the rat kidney. J. Pharmacol. Exp. Ther. 1990;255:1309-1313.

12 - Fernandes, M.H., Pestana, M. & Soares-da-Silva, P. Deamination of newly-formed dopamine in rat renal tissues. Br. J. Pharmacol. 1991;102:778-782.

13 - Soares-da-Silva, P., Fernandes, M.H. & Vieira-Coelho, M.A. In vivo effects of the monoamine oxidase inhibitors Ro 41-1049 and Ro 19-6327 on the production and fate of renal dopamine. J. Neural Trans. 1993 "in press".

14 - Fernandes MH and Soares-da-Silva P: Type A and B monoamine oxidase activities in the human and rat kidney. Acta Physiol. Scand. 1992;145:363-367.

15 - Soares-da-Silva, P. & Garrett, M.C. A study of the effects of tryptophan hydroxylase inhibition on 5-hydroxytryptamine and 5-hydroxyindolacetic acid (5-HIAA) levels in the brain of the rat: Implications for the origin of 5-HIAA. Mol. Neuropharmacol. 1991;1:83-90.

16 - Trendelenburg, U. The extraneuronal uptake and metabolism of catecholamines. In Catecholamines, ed. by Trendelenburg, U. & Weiner, N., Vol. 1, pp.279-319, Springer-Verlag, Berlin, 1988.

17 - Soares-da-Silva, P. & Fernandes, M.H. Regulation of dopamine synthesis in the rat kidney. J. Auton. Pharmacol. 1990;10 (Suppl. 1):s25-s30.

18 - Chan, Y.L. Cellular mechanisms of renal tubular transport of L-DOPA and its derivatives in the rat: microperfusions studies. J Pharmacol Exp Ther 1974;199:17-24.

Footnotes.

1 The present work was supported by a grant from the INIC (FmP1)

2 Permanent address: Faculty of Medical Dentistry, 4200 Porto, Portugal.

Regulation of Transcellular Transport by Dopamine Production in the Proximal Tubule

A.D. Baines, P. Ho, A. Debska-Slizien and
R. Drangova

Department of Clinical Biochemistry, The University of Toronto,
Toronto, Ontario, Canada M5G 1L5

ABSTRACT

Inhibiting aromatic amino acid decarboxylase with carbidopa reveals dopamine's links to Na and P homeostasis. Carbidopa increased by 20% the number of NaK-ATPase units associated with proximal tubular basolateral membranes (BLM) over a 4 hour period. SCH23390 also increased NaK-ATPase. The association of increased NaK-ATPase with the cytoskeleton was confirmed by finding that carbidopa increased triton-insoluble and decreased triton-soluble NaK-ATPase in LLC-PK cells. Carbidopa did not increase NaK-ATPase in rats fed a low salt diet. Adding DOPA to the diet restored the carbidopa response in salt depleted rats. Carbidopa increased brush border proton-antiporter activity in salt loaded rats but not in salt deprived rats. DA excretion increased from 1.9 to 2.8 nmol/d when dietary phosphate was increased from 0.03% to 0.7%. Reducing Ca intake from 0.7% to 0.017% increased DA excretion to 3.3 nmol/d. Inhibiting DA production with carbidopa decreased phosphate excretion. A low phosphate diet prevented the carbidopa induced increase of NaK-ATPase. Others have shown that SHR have defective linkage between DA_1 receptors and adenyl cyclase. Carbidopa did not stimulate NaK-ATPase in cortical BLM from SHR. Fractional phosphate excretion was higher and plasma phosphate is lower in SHR than in WKY. Carbidopa reduced phosphate excretion more in SHR than in WKY rats. In SHR rats endogenous DA regulates phosphate reabsorption through a system other than the defective DA_1-adenyl cyclase system in the S_1 segment. Further experiments are required to reveal the role of dopamine in abnormal Ca, P, Na and proton excretion by kidneys of hypertensive animals.

DOPAMINE AND SODIUM

One of the exquisite mysteries of epithelial transport is the subtle flow of information between apical and basolateral membranes that synchronizes solute entry and exit across the cell while maintaining a constant cell volume and internal environment. Dopamine is ideally situated to participate as an intermediary in the cross-talk between apical and basolateral membranes of the proximal tubule. It is generally accepted that dopamine inhibits both entry and exit steps for sodium and dopamine production is controlled by sodium intake. Dopamine also controls phosphate entry into the cell and dopamine production is controlled by phosphate intake. In this review we will examine the connections of dopamine, first to sodium, then to phosphate and finally to altered sodium and phosphate transport in spontaneously hypertensive rats (SHR).

There are three major control points for dopamine production and excretion. These are: circulating DOPA concentration, AAADC activity and dopamine secretion. Circulating DOPA, the main source of urinary dopamine (1,2), may (3) or may not (4) increase with salt intake. Entry of DOPA through peritubular and luminal surfaces may be sodium dependent (5). The V_{max} for aromatic amino acid decarboxylase, which converts DOPA to dopamine, is increased by a high salt intake (4,6,7). Dopamine is excreted primarily through the luminal membranes (1,2,8-10) by a process linked to proton transport and indirectly to sodium transport. Dopamine that escapes into the peritubular fluid is transported back into the cell through a mechanism that is sensitive to transmembrane potential (unpublished observations). Dopamine is metabolized by COMT and MAO in the proximal tubule (9) but salt intake does not appear to alter the degradation rate of dopamine (4,6). Dopamine content of cortical tissue from chronically denervated rats does not change significantly with dietary salt intake although dopamine excretion may increase 2 1/2 fold (4). In one study from our lab (11) dopamine content of denervated kidneys from rats eating a high salt diet was 4 ± 1 ng/g and in kidneys from low salt rats was 2 ± 1 ng/g. In another study (2) the values were 3 ± 0.5 and 3 ± 0.5. Hayashi (4) reported dopamine levels of 3.9 ± 0.7 in denervated kidneys from rats eating a high salt diet and 5.5 ± 2.0 ng/g in kidneys from rats eating a low salt diet. Constant internal dopamine concentration is consistent with the rapid turnover of DOPA to dopamine shown by micropuncture experiments (1,9). Increased dopamine excretion following protein ingestion results from increased DOPA (12). Increased dopamine excretion following salt intake results from an increased V_{max} for AAADC and possibly from increased DOPA concentration and dopamine secretion (3,4,6).

Why some hypertensive patients do not increases dopamine production following a protein meal is unknown (12). The answer, which may relate to defects in cellular DOPA uptake or decarboxylase activity (13,14) will help us understand the kidneys' role in the pathogenesis of hypertension.

The role of dopamine production in sodium transport was examined by using carbidopa to inhibit dopamine production. Within 4 hours after administering carbidopa the mass of NaK-ATPase associated with the basolateral membrane of proximal tubules increased by 15-20% as shown by

Western blotting with antibodies to the rat α-subunit of NaK-ATPase. V_{max} also increases but K_m for sodium or potassium or ouabain was unchanged (15). This effect was reproduced in basolateral membranes from proximal tubules isolated in a percoll gradient and was not seen in the outer medulla. A similar increase in BLM NaK-ATPase was produced by administration of SCH23390 18 hours previously. Inhibition of dopamine production or prolonged blockade of DA_1 receptors reveals that dopamine normally holds proximal tubular NaK-ATPase below its maximum activity in basolateral membranes. This sustained effect of endogenous low concentrations of dopamine acting on DA_1 receptors is different from the rapid onset of inhibition mediated by combined DA_1 and DA_2 receptors at higher concentrations of exogenous dopamine (16).

To confirm the effect of carbidopa on NaK-ATPase binding to the cytoskeleton we used an approached devised by Nelson and his colleagues (17). They found that triton-insoluble NaK-ATPase is associated with ankyrin and fodrin in basolateral membranes of cultured renal epithelial cells. The membrane associated form of NaK-ATPase (triton-insoluble) increased and the triton-soluble form decreased when cells become confluent. In their experiments NaK-ATPase associated with basolateral membranes increased because its residence time was prolonged. We have incubated confluent LLC-PK cells 3 and 8 days after seeding in DMEM/F12 medium with 10^5 M carbidopa for 18 hours. In cells exposed to carbidopa, triton-insoluble NaK-ATPase increased $13\pm2\%$ (S.E.; n=17; p<0.001) while the triton-soluble material decreased by $13\pm6\%$ (n=13; p=0.03).

A low salt diet increased basal NaK-ATPase activity and completely blocked the rise in NaK-ATPase in carbidopa treated rats (15). Adding excess dietary DOPA lowered basal NaK-ATPase and restored the response to carbidopa. Carbidopa had no effect on Na-H antiporter or Na-P cotransporter activity in brush border membranes vesicles from Wistar rats fed a normal salt diet. However we have found a small increase in amiloride inhibitable antiporter activity in brush border membrane vesicles from Sprague-Dawley rats fed an 8% salt diet for 7 days (unpublished observations). The effect of carbidopa in brush border membrane vesicles from rats fed a low salt diet was not significant. This suggests that endogenous dopamine may regulate NaK-ATPase by its effect on Na entry through the luminal proton antiporter (15).

The connection between dopamine and NaK-ATPase could be direct, through second messengers, to factors that regulate NaK-ATPase residence time in the basolateral membrane or indirect through factors that regulate sodium entry into the cell. Regulation of NaK-ATPase by sodium entry has been shown in cortical collecting tubules (18,19). Direct regulation of NaK-ATPase is suggested by analogy with PTH (20) which inhibits NaK-ATPase without evident effects on brush border function. The analogy with PTH is suggested by the fact that both dopamine and PTH inhibit brush border proton antiporter and phosphate cotransporter and both appear to inhibit basolateral membrane NaK-ATPase. Further experiments are required to establish the mechanisms by which dopamine controls the turnover of NaK-ATPase associated with the basolateral membrane cytoskeleton.

DOPAMINE AND PHOSPHATE

Observations similar to those which are used to designate dopamine as the proximal tubular natriuretic hormone, also reveal dopamine to be a phosphaturic paracrine hormone.

Exogenous dopamine is a potent phosphaturic agent (21-23) even when it has no natriuretic effect (21,23). Exogenously administered dopamine acts synergistically with exogenous PTH to increase phosphate excretion by phosphate depleted rats that are insensitive to either dopamine or PTH alone (22). Phosphate intake and dopamine excretion correlate (Fig 1) (24). Dopamine excretion increased within 1 day after increasing dietary phosphate. Reducing calcium content of a 0.7% phosphate diet from 0.7% to 0.017% stimulates both phosphate and dopamine excretion still further (Fig 1). Lowering calcium intake stimulates PTH secretion therefore these preliminary results suggest a connection between PTH and dopamine excretion. Where and how calcium and phosphate regulates dopamine excretion is not known.

The strong association between phosphate excretion and dopamine excretion suggests that sodium and phosphate cotransport into the cell could be a factor in the regulation of NaK-ATPase. The brush border phosphate cotransporter in Sprague-Dawley rats is inhibited by dopamine (23) presumably by a mechanism involving DA_1 receptors and adenyl cyclase. A role for dopamine regulation of phosphate and sodium transport is suggested by our observation that a low phosphate diet for 5 days completely prevented the usual NaK-ATPase increase that follows carbidopa treatment (submitted for publication). Clearance measurements, under inactin anesthesia, revealed that 18 hours after the first injection of carbidopa there was no difference in inulin clearance or fractional sodium excretion compared with untreated controls but fractional phosphate excretion was lower in carbidopa treated Wistar rats. Renal nerves had been removed 7 days previously therefore they were not involved in this response.

DOPAMINE AND SHR

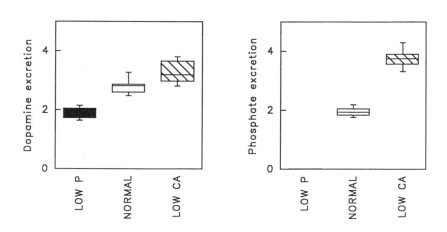

Fig 1. Box plot of phosphate (mmol/d) and dopamine (µg/d) excretion by Wistar rats fed either a low phosphate normal calcium diet (0.03% P, 0.7% Ca; LOW P) or a normal diet (0.7% P, 0.7% Ca; NORMAL) or a normal phosphate low calcium diet (0.7% P, 0.017% Ca; LOW CA) for 5 days. Box contains 25 to 75 percentiles; bars indicate 10th and 90th percentiles. Phosphate excretion by the LOW P group was too small to appear on the scale of this graph (0.006±0.003 mmol/d).

The proximal tubular antiporter in SHR rats is insensitive to dopamine (25) because of a defect in coupling of the DA_1 receptor to adenyl cyclase (26). Dopamine linkage to phospholipase C is also impaired in SHR (27). NaK-ATPase in the SHR basolateral membranes does not respond to inhibition of dopamine production with carbidopa (28). The lack of responsiveness to carbidopa in SHR is consistent with either a defect in dopamine linkage to adenyl cyclase or to phospholipase C linkage (27).

Defective coupling of DA_1 receptors and adenyl cyclase in SHR rats could make them insensitive to regulation of phosphate reabsorption by dopamine. To test this possibility we examined the effect of carbidopa on phosphate excretion and basolateral membrane NaK-ATPase in WKY and SHR rats (28). Clearance measurements, under inactin anesthesia, revealed that 18 hours after the first injection of carbidopa there was no difference in inulin clearance or fractional sodium excretion compared with untreated controls but fractional phosphate excretion was lower in the carbidopa treated SHR ($8.3\pm1.9\%$ vs $2.7\pm0.9\%$; $p=0.004$) as well as in the WKY rats (4.6 ± 0.9 and 2.5 ± 0.8). Under control conditions fractional phosphate excretion by SHR rats was higher than by WKY rats. Carbidopa lowered fractional excretion more in SHR than in WKY.

SUMMARY

Carbidopa was used to explore the role of endogenous dopamine production in the regulation of transcellular transport of sodium and phosphate. The results indicate that, in rats fed a normal salt and phosphate diet, endogenous dopamine restrains sodium and phosphate entry into the cell and the number of NaK-ATPase units associated with basolateral membranes. This restraining influence is not evident when rats are fed either a low phosphate or a low sodium diet. Dopamine production could be a significant factor in renal homeostatic response to high salt or phosphate diets.

Regulation of NaK-ATPase by endogenous dopamine, which involves DA_1 receptors in the proximal tubule, is lacking in SHR rats. These rats are mildly acidotic which could be evidence of abnormal proton antiporter regulation (29). Despite this evidence of defective DA_1 function in SHR rats endogenous dopamine regulates phosphate reabsorption in SHR. This unexpected observation suggests that the endogenous dopamine inhibits phosphate reabsorption in SHR by acting through a receptor other than the defective DA_1 receptor.

ACKNOWLEDGMENTS

This work was supported by grants from the Medical Research Council of Canada and the Kidney Foundation of Canada.

REFERENCES

1. Baines, A.D., Sole, M. and Chan, W. Production of urine free dopamine from plasma DOPA: a micropuncture study. Life Sci. 1980;26: 253-259.

2. Baines, A.D. and Drangova, R. Dopamine production by the isolated perfused rat kidney. Can J Physiol Pharmacol. 1984;62: 272-276.

3. Grossman, E., Hoffman, A., Chang, P.C., Keiser, H.R. and Goldstein, D.S. Increased spillover of dopa into arterial blood during dietary salt loading. Clin Sci. 1990;78: 423-429.

4. Hayashi, M., Yamaji, Y., Kitajima, Y. and Saruta, T. Effects of high salt intake on dopamine production in rat kidney. Am J Physiol. 1991;260: E675-E679.

5. Soares-da-Silva, P. and Fernandes, M.H. Sodium-dependence and ouabain-sensitivity of the synthesis of dopamine in renal tissues of the rat. Br J Pharmacol. 1992;105: 811-816.

6. Seri, I., Kone, B.C., Gullans, S.R., Aperia, A., Brenner, B.M. and Ballermann, B.J. Influence of Na^+ intake on dopamine-induced inhibition of renal cortical Na^+-K^+-ATPase. Am J Physiol. 1990;258: F52-F60.

7. Hayashi, M., Yamaji, Y., Kitajima, W. and Saruta, T. Aromatic L-amino acid decarboxylase activity along the rat nephron. Am J Physiol. 1990;258: F28-F33.

8. Suzuki, H., Nakane, H., Kawamura, M., Yoshizawa, M., Takeshita, E. and Saruta, T. Excretion and metabolism of dopa and dopamine by isolated perfused rat kidney. Am J Physiol. 1984;247: E285-E290.

9. Baines, A.D., Craan, A., Chan, W. and Morgunov, N. Tubular secretion and metabolism of dopamine, norepinephrine, methoxytyramine and normetanephrine by the rat kidney. J Pharmacol Exp Ther. 1979;208: 144-147.

10. Chan, Y.L. Cellular mechanisms of renal tubular transport of L-DOPA and its derivatives in the rat: microperfusion studies. J Pharmacol Exp Ther. 1976;199: 17-24.

11. Baines, A.D. Effects of salt intake and renal denervation on catecholamine catabolism and excretion. Kidney Intern. 1982;21: 316-322.

12. Clark, B.A., Rosa, R.M., Epstein, F.H., Young, J.B. and Landsberg, L. Altered dopaminergic responses in hypertension. Hypertension. 1992;19: 589-594.

13. Kuchel, O. and Shigetomi, S. Defective dopamine generation from dihydroxyphenylalanine in stale essential hypertensive patients. Hypertension. 1992;19: 634-638.

14. Gill, J.R., Jr., Grossman, E. and Goldstein, D.S. High urinary dopa and low urinary dopamine-to-dopa ratio in salt-sensitive hypertension. Hypertension. 1991;18: 614-621.

15. Baines, A.D., Ho, P. and Drangova, R. Proximal tubular dopamine production regulates basolateral Na-K-ATPase. Am J Physiol Renal,Fluid Electrolyte Physiol. 1992;262: F566-F571.

16. Bertorello, A. and Aperia, A. Both DA1 and DA2 receptor agonists are necessary to inhibit NaKATPase activity in proximal tubules from rat kidney. Acta Physiol Scand. 1988;132: 441-443.

17. Hammerton, R.W., Krzeminski, K.A., Mays, R.W., Ryan, T.A., Wollner, D.A. and Nelson, W.J. Mechanism for regulating cell surface distribution of Na^+, K^+-ATPase in polarized epithelial cells. Science. 1991;254: 847-850.

18. Barlet-Bas, C., Khadouri, C., Marsy, S. and Doucet, A. Enhanced intracellular sodium concentration in kidney cells recruits a latent pool of Na-K-ATPase whose size is modulated by corticosteroids. J Biol Chem. 1990;265: 7799-7803.

19. Blot-Chabaud, M., Wanstok, F., Bonvalet, J.-P. and Farman, N. Cell sodium-induced recruitment of Na^+-K^+-ATPase pumps in rabbit cortical collecting tubules is aldosterone-dependent. J Biol Chem. 1990;265: 11676-11681.

20. Ribeiro, C.P. and Mandel, L.J. Parathyroid hormone inhibits proximal tubule Na^+-K^+- ATPase activity. Am J Physiol Renal,Fluid Electrolyte Physiol. 1992;262: F209-F216.

21. Cuche, J.L., Marchand, G.R., Greger, R.F., Lang, F.C. and Knox, F.G. Phosphaturic effects of dopamine in dogs. Possible role of intrarenally produced dopamine on phosphate regulation. J Clin Invest. 1976;58: 71-76.

22. Issac, J., Berndt, T.J., Chinnow, S.L., Tyce, G.M., Dousa, T.P. and Knox, F.G. Dopamine enhances the phosphaturic response to parathyroid homone in phosphate-deprived rats. J Am Soc Nephrol. 1992;2: 1423-1429.

23. Isaac, J., Glahn, R.P., Appel, M.A., Onsgard, M., Dousa, T.P. and Knox, F.G. Mechanism of dopamine inhibition of renal phsophate transport. J Am Soc Nephrol. 1992;2: 1601-1607.

24. Berndt, T.J., Walakonis, R., MacDonald, A., Dousa, T.P., Tyce, G.M. and Knox, F.G. Increased dietary phosphate intake increases urinary dopamine excretion. J Am Soc Nephrol. 1990;1: 575.

25. Gesek, F.A. and Schoolwerth, A.C. Hormone responses of proximal Na^+-H^+ exchanger in spontaneously hypertensive rats. Am J Physiol. 1991;261: F526-F536.

26. Kinoshita, S., Sidhu, A. and Felder, R.A. Defective dopamine-1 receptor adenylate cyclase coupling in the proximal convoluted tubule from the spontaneously hypertensive rat. J Clin Invest. 1989;84: 1849-1856.

27. Chen, C.-J., Vyas, S.J., Eichberg, J. and Lokhandwala, M.F. Diminished phospholipase C activation by dopamine in spontaneously hypertensive rats. Hypertension. 1992;19: 102-108.

28. Baines, A.D., Ho, P. and Drangova, R. Regulation of NaK-ATPase by dopamine produced in proximal tubules is absent in SHR rats. J Am Soc Nephrol. 1991;2: 424.

29. Lucas, P.A., Lacour, B., Comte, L. and Dr:ueke, T. Pathogenesis of abnormal acid-base balance in the young spontaneously hypertensive rat. Clinical Science. 1988;75: 29-34.

Studies on the Tubular Cell Outward Dopamine Transport in the Rat Kidney[1]

P. Soares-da-Silva and M. Pestana[2]

Department of Pharmacology and Therapeutics, Faculty of
Medicine, 4200 Porto, Portugal

ABSTRACT

The present study has determined the kinetic characteristics of the outflow of dopamine of renal origin in slices of rat renal cortex loaded with exogenous L-dihydroxyphenylalanine (L-DOPA, 5 to 5000 µM). The application of the Michaelis-Menten equation to the net transport of newly-formed dopamine has allowed the identification of a saturable (carrier-mediated transfer) and a non-saturable component (diffusion). The V_{max} (nmol g^{-1} 15 min^{-1}) and K_m (nM) values for the saturable component were, respectively, 340±41 and 396±45. Up to a concentration of 250 nmol g^{-1} of dopamine the non-saturable component was found not to play an important role. The results of perifusion studies suggest that a considerable amount of released dopamine from tubular epithelial cells is taken up into a monoamine oxidase (MAO) enriched cellular compartment, before appearing in the effluent. In conclusion, it is suggested that the newly-formed dopamine in tubular epithelial cells is transported out of this compartment by a carrier-mediated transport system. A considerable amount of the released dopamine appears to be taken up into a MAO enriched compartment shortly after being released; this sequence of events might constitute an important mechanism for the inactivation of the amine.

INTRODUCTION

In various animal species, the proximal nephron has been shown to produce dopamine from DOPA present in the tubular filtrate and the locally formed amine demonstrated to activate specific receptors distributed to this renal area. The activation of type D_1 dopamine receptors located in tubular epithelial cells produces a decreased tubular reabsorption of sodium (1), most probably as a result of inhibition of both the Na^+-K^+ ATPase and the Na^+-H^+ exchanger (2, 3). On the other hand, Na^+ and the mechanisms regulating the tubular transport of Na^+ have been found of some importance in the control of dopamine synthesis in renal tissues (4, 5). Furthermore, there is evidence to suggest that the locally formed dopamine may act in a cell-to-cell manner, as a paracrine or autocrine substance, since the cells which convert DOPA to dopamine contain or are near those endowed with D_1 receptors (6, 7).

© 1993 Pergamon Press Ltd.
Printed in Great Britain.

In order to be active, the dopamine with origin in tubular epithelilal cells, is, however, expected to leave the cellular compartment where the synthesis has occurred and once outside the cell to be able to activate the dopamine receptors located in the extracellular surface of cell membrane (8). It has not been clarified till now whether there is a preferential cell outward transport of dopamine at the basolateral or the apical cell borders. Indirect evidence, however, supports the view that dopamine can leave the tubular cell by the apical and basolateral borders, although the basolateral one may be particularly important under physiological conditions. The apical cell border has been demonstrated not to take up dopamine from the tubular fluid (9), whereas the basolateral one has been implicated in the process of active secretion of catecholamines, including dopamine, present in the interstitial medium (10). This brings into discussion the question of whether and to which extent is the dopamine produced in tubular epithelial cells submitted to an uptake process after being released into the extracellular medium (inside-outside cell recirculation); this is most likely to occur at the basolateral cell border considering the diminute ability of the apical cell border to take up the amine. In case it might occur, the inside-outside cell recirculation of newly-formed dopamine is expected to play a role in the renal handling of the amine. This would constitute a way to stabelize the levels of the amine in the extracellular medium, but, on the other hand, would favour the inactivation of the amine. In fact, renal tissues are endowed with one of the highest MAO activities in the body (11) and deamination of newly-formed dopamine into 3,4-dihydroxyphenylacetic acid (DOPAC) represents a major pathway for the inactivation of the amine (12, 13).

The present work has examined the presence of an active transport system for dopamine, determined the kinetic characteristics of the outflow of dopamine of renal origin and evaluated the question of the fate of the amine after being released into the extracellular medium.

MATERIALS and METHODS

Male Wistar rats (Biotério do Instituto Gulbenkian de Ciência, Oeiras, Portugal) 45-60 days old and weighing 200-250 g were used in the experiments. Animals were sacrificed by decapitation under ether anesthesia and both kidneys removed and rinsed free from blood with saline (NaCl 0.9%). The kidneys were then placed on an ice cold glass plate, the kidney poles removed and slices of the renal cortex approximately 0.5 mm thick and weighing about 25 mg wet weight were prepared with a scalpel. Thereafter, renal slices were preincubated for 30 min in 2 ml gassed (95% O_2 and 5% CO_2) and warm (37ºC) Krebs' solution. The Krebs' solution had the following composition (mM): NaCl 120, · KCl 4.7, CaCl$_2$ 2.4, MgSO$_4$ 1.2, KH$_2$PO$_4$ 1.2,

NAHCO$_3$ 25, EDTA 0.4 and glucose 11; l-alpha-methyl-p-tyrosine (50 µM), tropolone (50 µM) and copper sulphate (10 µM) were also added to the Krebs' solution in order to inhibit the enzymes tyrosine hydroxylase and catechol-O-methyltransferase and inhibit the endogenous inhibitors of dopamine ß-hydroxylase, respectively. In some experiments, inhibition of MAO was performed by adding pargyline (100 µM) to the medium. After preincubation, renal slices were incubated for 15 min in Krebs' solution with added L-DOPA. The preincubation and incubation were carried out in glass test tubes, continuously shaken throughout the experiment.

In the experiments performed with the aim of determine the presence and characterize the kinetic parametters of the outward transport mechanism for dopamine in renal slices, tissues were loaded with increasing concentrations (5 to 5000 µM) of L-DOPA for 15 min and the amount of newly-formed dopamine accumulated in the tissue and that which has escaped into the incubation medium determined; up to a concentration of 5000 µM L-DOPA, the pH of the incubation medium remained stable at 7.4. This set of experiments was performed in conditions of MAO inhibition. K_m and V_{max} values for the outward transport of newly-formed dopamine were calculated from linear regression analysis; the substrate transported (nmoles of dopamine present in the incubation medium) was plotted against the product of the division between the susbtrate transported by the concentration of dopamine to be transported (nmoles of total dopamine formed, obtained from the algebraic sum of the amount accumulated in the tissue plus that present in the incubation medium). In these experimental conditions, the movement of newly-formed dopamine is expected to be mainly from the intracellular to the extracellular medium; however, it may be hypothetized that the net transfer of dopamine would involve a carrier-mediated transport, but diffusion may also contribute to total transfer. The determination of carrier transport and diffusion in this experimental model was performed as defined by Neame & Richards (14) with the utilization of the expression

$$(V_{max}.[S]/[S]+K_m)+(K_d.[S])$$
$$(\text{carrier transport})+(\text{diffusion})$$

where [S] is the concentration of the substrate to be transported and K_d the diffusion constant. Values for K_m and V_{max} were obtained by the method above described.

In another series of experiments, slices of rat renal cortex were incubated for 15 min in warm and gassed 2 ml Krebs' solution with added L-DOPA (100 µM) in the presence or the absence of pargyline (100 µM). At the end of incubation the tissues were collected and immediatly placed in glass perifusion chambers and perifused with warm and gassed Krebs' solution at a rate of 350 µl min^{-1} by means of a Gilson pump (Minipulse 2). After allowing a 30 min stabilization period, five consecutive 10 min perifusate samples were collected into glass tubes kept on ice and containing 500µl of

2 M perchloric acid. At the end of the perifusion, the kidney fragments were collected, blotted with filter paper and placed in 2 ml of 0.2 M perchloric acid. The levels (in nmol g⁻¹ 10 min⁻¹) of dopamine and DOPAC in the perifusate were logarithmically transformed, plotted against the time of perifusion and the slope of decline calculated using linear regression analysis. The constant rates of amine and amine metabolite in the outflow (k) were then obtained from the expression, k=slope value/0.434 (15). The fractional outflow was obtained by dividing the amount of dopamine and DOPAC in the perifusate (nmol g⁻¹ 10 min⁻¹) by the tissue content of dopamine and DOPAC (nmol g⁻¹).

The assay of dopamine and DOPAC in kidney slices and samples of the incubation medium or the perifusate was performed by means of high pressure liquid chromatography with electrochemical detection, as previously described (17). The lower limit for detection of dopamine and DOPAC were, respectively, 500 and 750 fmol 50 µl⁻¹.

RESULTS

The production of dopamine was found to be dependent on the concentration of L-DOPA used and reached its maximum at 2500 µM L-DOPA (see also reference 12). A considerable amount of the total dopamine formed from added L-DOPA in kidney slices (more than 50%) was found to escape into the incubation medium. The application of the Michaelis-Menten equation to the net transport of newly-formed dopamine has allowed the identification of a saturable (carrier-mediated transfer) and a non-saturable component (diffusion). In figure 1 are shown the two components of dopamine transport and the total rate of amine transfer, as a plot of the amount of dopamine which has escaped into the incubation medium (rate of transport) against the total amount of dopamine formed (substrate concentration) in rat kidney slices. The corresponding Eadie-Hofstee plot of the saturable component is also shown (figure 1). The V_{max} (nmol g⁻¹ 15 min⁻¹) and K_m (nM) values for the saturable component were, respectively, 340±41 and 396±45. Diffusion appears to be of some importance only when the amount of dopamine to be transported exceeds 250 nmol g⁻¹.

The results obtained in perifusion experiments show that the levels of newly-formed dopamine and DOPAC in the perifusate progressively decreased along the perifusion period, being the constant rate of loss for the amine (k=0.044±0.004) significantly higher in comparison with that for the deaminated metabolite DOPAC (k=0.029±0.003). The fractional outflow of DOPAC was found to be significantly higher than that for dopamine and did not tend to decrease throughout the perifusion period, as was observed for the amine (figure 2); this resulted in that the proportion of

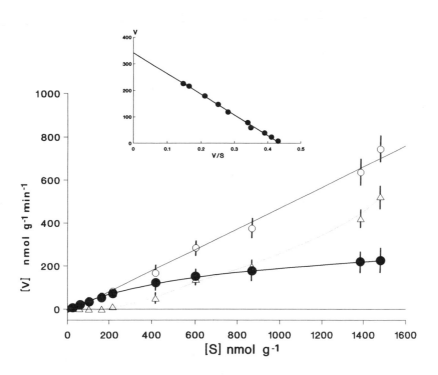

Figure 1. Outward transfer of newly-formed dopamine in slices of rat renal cortex incubated with increasing concentrations of L-DOPA (5 to 5000 μM) for 15 min. The results are on the the two components of dopamine transfer, saturable (closed circles) and non-saturable (open triangles), and the total rate of amine transfer (open circles), as a plot of the amount of dopamine which has escaped into the incubation medium (rate of amine transport; [V], in nmol g-1 15 min-1) against the total amount of dopamine formed (substrate concentration; [S], in nmol g-1) in the rat kidney slices. *Inset*: Eadie-Hofstee plot of the saturable component of newly-formed outward transfer in slices of rat renal cortex incubated with increasing concentrations of L-DOPA (5 to 5000 μM) for 15 min. The V_{max} (nmol g-1 15 min-1) and K_m (nM) values for the saturable component were, respectively, 340±41 and 396±45.

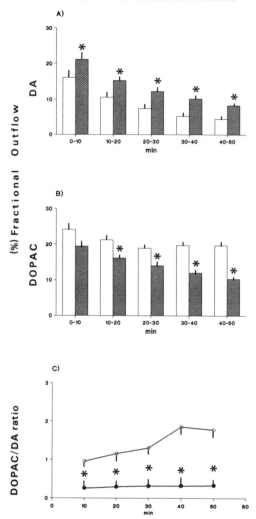

Figure 2.   Fractional outflow of (A) dopamine and (B) DOPAC in five consecutive 10 min perifusate samples of rat cortical slices previously loaded with 100 µM L-DOPA; the results shown are on the observations for the fractional outflow in control conditions (open columns) and in the presence of pargyline (100 µM; hatched columns). The lower part of the figure (C) shows the results on the DOPAC/dopamine ratios in perifusate along the 50 min perifusion period in control conditions (open circles) and in the presence of pargyline (100 µM; closed circles). Each column or point represents the mean of 7 to 8 experiments per group; vertical lines show SEM. Significantly different from corresponding controls (P<0.01) using the Student's "t" test.

DOPAC to dopamine in the perifusate progressively increased throughout the perifusion period from 0.95 ± 0.07 to 1.77 ± 0.25 (figure 2). In addition, the DOPAC/dopamine ratio in the perifusate was found to be 3-fold higher than that in the tissues. Pargyline (100 µM), produced a marked decrease (44%-54% reduction) in the outflow levels and in the fractional outflow of DOPAC and significantly increased the levels of dopamine in the effluent (100 to 150% increase) and the fractional outflow of dopamine (figure 2a). However, the constant rates of loss for both dopamine ($k=0.039\pm0.002$) and DOPAC ($k=0.033\pm0.001$) were similar to those of controls. In conditions of MAO inhibition, in contrast with that observed in controls, the proportion of DOPAC to dopamine in the perifusate was similar to that found in the tissues and only slightly increased from 0.26 ± 0.02 to 0.33 ± 0.02 throughout the perifusion period (figure 2b).

DISCUSSION

The results presented here demonstrate that the outflow of newly-formed dopamine in kidney slices loaded with exogenous L-DOPA follows a Michaelis-Menten kinetics with a saturable component and a non-saturable one, the latter assuming particular importance only at higher concentrations of the substrate. The analysis of the outflow of dopamine and DOPAC revealed a significantly higher fractional outflow of DOPAC in comparison with that for dopamine, suggesting that dopamine exiting from tubular epithelial cells is a constant source for deamination into DOPAC. The finding that the proportion of DOPAC to dopamine in the overflow was 3-fold that in the tissues and progressively increased throughout the perifusion period, suggests that dopamine before reaching the perifusion medium may cross a MAO enriched cellular compartment. The finding that the levels of newly-formed dopamine and DOPAC in the outflow follow a monoexponential pattern of decay appears to be consistent with the view that both dopamine and DOPAC are derived from a single cellular compartment. This suggestion is further stressed by the result showing similar constant rates of loss for both compounds in control conditions and during MAO inhibition, in spite of the changes in dopamine and DOPAC outflow levels.

In kidney, the deamination of newly-formed dopamine is rather unlikely to occur in a neuronal compartment. Firstly, both type A and B MAO have been demonstrated to be mainly located in non-neuronal tissues (16, 17). Secondly, it has been suggested that the dopamine formed in renal tissues loaded with L-DOPA has most probably no access to nerve terminals, as evidenced by the finding that the levels of noradrenaline in kidney slices did not change when up to 2500 µM L-DOPA is added to the incubation medium (12). Taken together, these results support the view that newly-formed dopamine in kidney slices is not taken up to sympathetic nerve terminals, being instead mainly deaminated in an extraneuronal compartment.

The data presented here appears to suggests that dopamine, before reaching the perifusion fluid, is intensely deaminated into DOPAC. This suggestion is supported by the findings that the proportion of DOPAC to dopamine in the perifusate is significantly higher than that in the tissues (0.95 vs 0.30) and DOPAC/dopamine ratios in the perifusate progressivelly increased throughout the perifusion period. Another result supporting this view is that the fractional outflow of DOPAC was significantly higher than that for dopamine and did not tend to decrease along the perifusion period, as was observed for dopamine. Altogether, these results would favour the possibility that dopamine produced in tubular epithelial cells after being released into the extracellular medium might be submitted to an uptake process into a MAO enriched celular compartment. The uptake process of the released dopamine is most likely to occur at the basolateral cell border, since the luminal border has been shown not to take up the amine (9), and appears to constitute an important mechanism for the inactivation of the released amine. The identification and kinetic characterization of the outward transport system for dopamine in renal tissues is of particular relevance, considering the evidence accumulated over the last years suggesting that dopamine with origin in tubular epithelial cells may have important physiological actions in the control of tubular reabsorption of sodium. The tubular actions of locally formed dopamine in the control of sodium reabsorption have been suggested to correspond to paracrine or autocrine effects due to the fact that the amine is believed to be produced in close proximity to the cells or by the cells in which the dopamine receptors are located.

CONCLUSION

It is suggested that the newly-formed dopamine in tubular epithelial cells is transported out of this compartment by a carrier-mediated transport system. A considerable amount of the released dopamine appears to be taken up into a MAO enriched compartment shortly after being released; this sequence of events might constitute an important mechanism for the inactivation of the amine.

REFERENCES

1 - Hedge, S.S., Ricci, A., Amenta, F. & Lokhandwala, M.F. Evidence from functional and autoradiographic studies for the presence of tubular dopamine-1

receptores and their involvement in the renal effects of fenoldopam. J. Pharmacol. Exp. Ther. 1989;251:1237-1245.

2 - Bertorello A, Hokfelt T, Goldstein M and Aperia A: Proximal tubule Na+-K+-ATPase activity is inhibited during high-salt diet: evidence for DA-mediated effect. Am. J. Physiol. 1988;254:F795-F801.

3 - Felder, C.C., Campbell, T., Albrecht, F. & Jose, P.A. Dopamine inhibits Na+-H+ exchanger activity in renal BBMV by stimulation of adenylate cyclase. Am. J. Physiol. 1990;259:F297-F303.

4 - Soares-da-Silva, P. & Fernandes, M.H. Inhibitory effects of guanosine 3':5'-cyclic monophosphate on the synthesis of dopamine in the rat kidney. Br. J. Pharmacol. 1991;103:1923-1927.

5 - Soares-da-Silva, P. & Fernandes, M.H. Sodium-dependence and ouabain-sensitivity of the synthesis of dopamine in renal tissues of the rat. Br. J. Pharmacol. 1992;105:811-816.

6 - Jose, P.A., Felder, R.A., Holloway, R.R. & Eisner, G.M. Dopamine receptors modulate sodium excretion in denervated kidney. Am. J. Physiol. 1986;250:F1033-F1038.

7 - Siragy, H.M., Felder, R.A., Howell, N.L., Chevalier, R.L., Peach, M.J. & Carey, R.M. Evidence that intrarenal dopamine dopamine acts as a paracrine susbtance at the renal tubule. Am. J. Physiol. 1989;257:F469-F477.

8 - Jose, P.A., Raymond, J.R., Bates, M.D., Aperia, A., Felder, R.A. & Carey, R.M. (1992). The renal dopamine receptors. J. Am. Soc. Nephrol. 1992;2:1265-1278.

9 - Chan, Y.L. Cellular mechanisms of renal tubular transport of L-DOPA and its derivatives in the rat: microperfusions studies. J. Pharmacol. Exp. Ther. 1976;199:17-24.

10 - Rennick, B.R. Renal tubule transport of organic cations. Am. J. Physiol. 1981;240:F83-F89.

11 - Kopin, I.J. Catecholamine metabolism: basic aspects and clinical significance. Pharmacol. Rev. 1985;37:333-364.

12 - Fernandes, M.H., Pestana, M. & Soares-da-Silva. P. Deamination of newly-formed dopamine in rat renal tissues. Br. J. Pharmacol. 1991;102:778-782.

13 - Fernandes, M.H. and Soares-da-Silva, P. Sequantial involvement of monoamine oxidase and catechol-O-methyltransferase in the metabolism of newly-formed dopamine in rat renal tissues. Advances in Biosciences (this volume).

14 - Neame, K.D. & Richards, T.G. Elementary kinetics of membrane carrier transport. Blackwell Scientific Publications. Oxford, 1972.

15 - Brodie, B.B., Costa, E., Dlabac, A., Neff, N.H. & Smookler, H.H. Application of steady state kinetics to the estimation of synthesis rate and turnover time of tissue catecholamines. J. Pharmacol. Exp. Ther. 1966;154:493-498.

16 - Caramona, M.M. & Soares-da-Silva, P. Evidence for an extraneuronal location of monoamine oxidase in renal tissues. Naunyn-Schmiedeberg's Arch. Pharmacol. 1990;341:411-413.

17 - Soares-da-Silva, P., Fernandes, M.H. Albino-Teixeira A., Azevedo, I. & Pestana, M. Brief transient ischemia induces long-term depletion of norepinephrine without affecting the aromatic amino acid decarboxylase and monoamine oxidase activities in the rat kidney. J. Pharmacol. Exp. Ther. 192;260:902-908.

Footnotes.

1 The present work was supported by a grant from the INIC (FmP1)

2 on leave from the Dept. of Nephrology, Faculty of Medicine, 4200 Porto, Portugal.

Molecular Biology of Dopamine Receptors: An Overview

Pedro A. Jose*, Robin A. Felder†,
Frederick J. Monsma, Jr‡, David R. Sibley‡ and
M. Maral Mouradian‡

*Department of Pediatrics, Georgetown University Children's
Medical Center, Washington, DC 20007, USA
†Department of Pathology, University of Virginia Center for the
Health Sciences, Charlottesville, VA 22908, USA
‡Experimental Therapeutics Branch, National Institute of
Neurological Disorders and Stroke, Bethesda, MD 20892, USA

ABSTRACT: Dopamine receptors in the brain have been classified into D_1 and D_2 subtypes, based on pharmacological data. However, five different dopamine receptors have now been identified using molecular biologic techniques. Two of the subtypes (D_{1A}, D_{1B} also known as D_5) are each coupled to the stimulation of adenylyl cyclase and correspond to the classically described D_1 receptor. The D_2, D_3, and D_4 receptors are coupled to the inhibition of adenylyl cyclase and correspond to the classically described D_2 receptor. A D_1 dopamine receptor linked to stimulation of phospholipase C activity has not yet been cloned. Outside the central nervous system, peripheral dopamine receptors have been classified into the DA_1 and DA_2 subtypes. The pharmacological properties of DA_1 receptors roughly approximate those of D_1 receptors, while those of DA_2 receptors approximate those of D_2 receptors. To date, all of the dopamine receptors cloned in brain are also expressed in tissues outside the central nervous system. For example, the D_{1A}, D_{1B}, and D_3 receptor genes are expressed in specific nephron segments. The D_4 receptor gene is expressed in the heart.

Dopamine is an endogenous catecholamine which modulates many physiological functions, including behavior, movement, nerve conduction, hormone synthesis and release, blood pressure, and ion fluxes. Dopamine receptors in the brain have been classified into D_1 and D_2 subtypes, based on pharmacological work in the 1970's (1). Several dopamine receptors have been purified to homogeneity (2,3,), and the genes/cDNA for several dopamine receptors have been cloned from brain (D_{1A}, D_{1B} also known as D_5, D_2, D_3, D_4) (Table 1a and 1b) and expressed in several mammalian host cell lines (4-19).

Table 1A. Dopamine receptors linked to the stimulation of adenylyl cyclase (adapted from ref 19).

Current nomenclature	D_1	D_5
Alternative nomenclature	D_{1A}	D_{1B}
Amino acids 　　Human 　　Rat	446 446	477 475
Introns in gene	Yes	No
Human chromosome	5	4
mRNA distribution 　　Brain 　　Kidney*	caudate-putamen, nucleus accumbens, olfactory tubercle proximal convoluted tubule, thick ascending limb of Henle	hippocampus, hypothalamus proximal convoluted tubule

Table 1B. Dopamine receptors linked to the inhibition of adenylyl cyclase (adapted from ref 19).

Current nomenclature	D_{2S}/D_{2L}	D_3	D_4
Alternative nomenclature	D_{2A-S}/D_{2A-L}	D_{2B}	D_{2C}
Amino Acids 　　Human 　　Rat	414/443 415/444	400 446	387 368
Introns in gene	Yes	Yes	Yes
Human chromosome	11	3	11
mRNA distribution 　　Brain 　　Kidney*	caudate-putamen, nucleus accumbens, olfactory tubercle glomerulus, proximal tubule	olfactory tubercle hypothalamus nucleus accumbens not specified	frontal cortex, medulla, midbrain not tested **

* complete mapping not available ** present in the heart

The D_{1A} and D_{1B} receptors correspond to the classically described "D_1" receptors that are linked to the stimulation of adenylyl cyclase, and to which D_1 antagonists (e.g.SCH 23390) and D_1 agonists (e.g. fenoldopam, SKF 38393) are bound with high affinity. While dopamine and D_1 agonists have a higher affinity to D_{1B} than D_{1A} receptors, they have similar affinities to D_1 antagonists (8,9). The D_{1A} (4-8) and D_{1B} (8-10) receptors interact with the guanine nucleotide binding protein, G_s to stimulate adenylyl cyclase. This results in the formation of cAMP which in turn binds to and activates protein kinase A (19-23). The D_2, D_3, and D_4 receptors correspond to the classically described "D_2" receptors that are linked to the inhibition of adenylyl cyclase (11,12,15,16). The "D_2" drugs (antagonists like YM-09151, spiperone and agonists like quinpirole) have similar affinities to the D_2, D_3, and D_4 receptors with some exceptions. For example, the rank order potency for clozapine affinities is $D_4 > D_2 > D_3$; spiroperidol is $D_2 > D_3 = D_4$; domperidone is $D_2 > D_3$; quinpirole is $D_3 > D_4 > D_2$. For dopamine the rank order affinity is $D_3 > D_{1B} > D_2 > D_4 > D_{1A}$. The pathway involved in the D_2 receptor-mediated inhibition of adenylyl cyclase is similar to that utilized for the D_1 receptor except that the D_2 receptor interacts with G_i. However, there appear to be other pathways involved in dopaminergic signal transduction. Depending upon the cellular milieu, D_2 receptors may increase or decrease intracellular calcium and phosphatidyl inositol hydrolysis (17). In addition, D_2 and D_3 receptors can activate K^+ channels in the brain (24) and the pituitary gland. We first described in the kidney a D_1 receptor capable of activating phosphatidyl inositol-specific phospholipase C leading to generation of inositol phosphates (and diacylglycerol), (25,26). This finding has been confirmed by others in the kidney (27), brain striatum (28), and the retina (29). However, this D_1 like receptor gene has not yet been cloned. There is preliminary evidence by cloning techniques of yet another dopamine receptor subtype different from the previously cloned dopamine receptors (30). Whether the latter receptor is linked to phosphatidyl inositol specific phospholipase C remains to be determined.

Dopamine receptors (like other related receptor proteins) have seven stretches of 20-26 hydrophobic amino acids which form putative transmembrane domains (21). The seven transmembrane domains are configured as amphipathic α-helices with charged residues facing inward forming a dopamine binding pocket and uncharged residues facing the membrane lipids. There are potential sites for N-linked glycosylation on the extracellular domains. The intracellular loops and the carboxy termini contain several sites for potential phosphorylation by various kinases such as protein kinase A and protein kinase C. Several intracellular regions close to the membrane are implicated for G protein coupling of these receptors. These regions comprise the carboxyl end of the second intracellular loop, the amino and carboxyl end of the third intracellular loop, and the amino portion of the carboxyl terminus (21,31). The third loop regions seem to be most important in conferring specificity of coupling to G proteins. The D_{1A} and D_{1B} dopamine receptors have small third cytoplasmic loops and long carboxy termini. This seems to be a characteristic of receptors that couple to G_s. The D_2, D_3, and D_4 receptors, on the other hand, have long third cytoplasmic loops and short carboxy termini, a characteristic of most, but not all, receptors that couple to G_i. By analogy with β-adrenergic receptors, some highly conserved residues may play important roles; highly conserved cysteines in the second and third extracellular loop may form a disulfide bond which stabilizes the binding pocket. In recent studies we have found that alkylation of sulfhydryl groups interfere with high affinity agonist binding sites (unpublished observations). Experiments using site-directed mutagenesis have uncovered sequences that are important in ligand binding and signal transduction. For example, aspartate 80 of the D_{2short} receptor is critical in conferring pH and sodium sensitivity to ligand binding (32). This residue may also play an important role in modulating adenylyl cyclase activity. Substitution of serine 202 with alanine in the 5th transmembrane domain of the D_{1A} receptor decreases affinity with agonists but not with antagonists; substitution of serine 199 with alanine decreases affinity to both agonists and antagonists (33).

The D_{1A} and D_{1B} receptor genes are encoded by a single exon (the D_{1A} receptor has an intron in the 5' untranslated region, 18). A D_{1B} pseudo-gene has also been reported (10). These receptors are highly homologous to one another (4-10). Thus, the D_{1A} receptor is approximately 50% identical at the amino acid level to the D_{1B} receptor. The D_2, D_3, and D_4 receptors are encoded by a mosaic of exons (11-14). These exons participate in an alternative splicing scheme which leads to expression of isoforms of the D_2 (termed D_{2long} and

D_{2short} based on the length of the cDNA) or D_3 receptor(12,34). Another D_2 receptor, different from the D_{2short} and D_{2long} has been described (35).

D_{1A}/D_2 interaction:

In Chinese hamster ovary cells expressing D_{1A} receptors, D_1 agonists do not affect arachidonic acid release. However, when both D_{1A} and D_2 receptors are co-expressed, activation of both subtypes results in a marked synergistic potentiation of arachidonic acid release (36). Felder et al also reported that the D_{2long} receptors transfected in Chinese hamster ovary cells potentiate arachidonic acid release by a mechanism involving protein kinase C and intracellular calcium but independent of the D_2 receptor's inhibition of adenylyl cyclase (37).

CLASSIFICATION OF RENAL DOPAMINE RECEPTORS:

Outside the central nervous system, Goldberg divided the dopamine receptors into the DA_1 and DA_2 subtypes, based on synaptic localization (38). The pharmacological properties of DA_1 receptors roughly approximate those of D_1 receptors, while those of DA_2 receptors approximate those of D_2 receptors (20-23).

LOCALIZATION OF RENAL DOPAMINE RECEPTORS:

Pharmacological methods: These methods have facilitated the localization of dopamine receptor subtypes to specific segments of the renal vasculature and the nephron (Table 1, ref 18, appendix A) (22-26). D_1 receptors have been identified in muscular layers of the main renal artery to the afferent arteriole. The highest density of D_1 receptors is found in brush border and basolateral membranes of proximal tubules (convoluted > straight); we have also solubilized D_1 receptors from this nephron segment (39-43). D_1 receptors are present in lesser quantities in the cortical collecting duct and least in medullary thick ascending limb of Henle (44-47). D_2-like receptors are also present in adventitial and endothelial cell layers of renal vessels (23). D_2 receptors predominate in glomeruli (43) although D_1 receptors become apparent in cultured mesangial cells. D_2 receptors are also present in the proximal tubule brush border and basolateral membranes (41). A D_2-like receptor called the DA_{2k} has also been described in inner medullary collecting duct cells (48).

Molecular biological methods: Except for the D_3 receptor, previous studies, including our own, have not detected dopamine receptor gene expression in the kidney using Northern blot analysis or polymerase chain reaction (PCR) using RNA obtained from whole kidney tissue (4-14). We have utilized ribonuclease protection assays and reverse transcriptase/PCR (RT/PCR) to detect expression of various dopamine receptor genes in specific nephron regions obtained by iron oxide and magnet, sieving and differential centrifugation (49-52). We found that the D_{1A}, D_{1B} and D_{2long}, are expressed in proximal tubules, medulla, and intrarenal arterial vessels.(49-52). A limitation of the sieving method is that 100% purity is not ensured. In order to eliminate any possible cross-contamination, we performed RT/PCR in microdissected nephron segments. We were able to detect D_{2long} receptor gene expression in glomeruli and D_{1A} receptor gene expression in the proximal convoluted tubule (confirmed by sequencing) but not in the cortical collecting duct although a D_1 receptor is also found in this segment by radioligand binding and biochemical studies (49-52). Thus, dopamine receptor genes may be selectively expressed in different nephron segments subserving specific regulatory roles on sodium transport. The first specific aim of this application will expand these studies and determine not only the type but also the quantity of dopamine receptor gene expressed in these nephron segments. In situ hybridization studies also suggest the presence of D_{1A} receptors in medullary thick ascending limb of Henle (53). We have cloned and expressed a dopamine receptor from rat renal proximal tubules (54) that is homologous to the D_{1B} receptor cloned from rat brain (8).

Since no novel "peripheral" dopamine receptor has thus far been cloned and since all of the dopamine receptors cloned in brain have been found to be expressed in tissues outside the central nervous system (14, 49-55), we suggest that the nomenclature for brain dopamine receptors be utilized for peripheral tissues as well.

REFERENCES:

1.   Kebabian, J.W, ,Calne, D.B. Multiple receptors for dopamine. Nature (Lond) 1979; 277: 93-96.

2.   Senogles, S.E., Amlaiky, N., Falardeau, P., Caron, MG. Purification of the D_2 dopamine receptor from bovine anterior pituitary. J Biol Chem .1988; 263: 18996-19002.

3.   Sidhu, A. Novel affinity purification of D-1 dopamine receptors from rat striatum. J Biol Chem. 1990; 265: 10065-10072.

4.   Dearry, A., Gingrich, J.A., Falardeau, P., Fremeau, R.T. Jr., Bates, M.D., Caron, M.G. Molecular cloning and expression of the gene for a human D_1 dopamine receptor. Nature (Lond). 1990; 347: 72-75.

5.   Monsma, F.J. Jr., Mahan, L.C., McVittie, L.D., Gerfen, C.R., Sibley, D.R. Molecular cloning and expression of a D_1 dopamine receptor linked to adenylyl cyclase activation. Proc Natl Acad Sci USA. 1990; 87: 6723-6727.

6.   Sunahara, R.K., Niznik, H.B., Weiner, D.M., Stormann, T.M., Brann, M.R., Kennedy, J.L., Gelernter, J.L., Rozmahel, R., Yang, Y., Israel, Y., Seeman, P., O'Dowd, B.F.   Human dopamine D_1 receptor encoded by an intronless gene on chromosome 5. Nature (Lond). 1990; 347: 80-83.

7.   Zhou, Q.Y., Grandy, D.K., Thambi, L., Kushner, J.A., Van Tol, H.H., Cone, R., Pribnow, D., Salon, J., Bunzow, J.R., Civelli, O. Cloning and expression of human and rat D_1 dopamine receptors. Nature (Lond). 1990; 347: 76-79.

8.   Tiberi, M., Jarvie, K.R., Silva, C., Bertrand, L., Yang-Feng, T.L., Fremeau, R.T. Jr., Caron, M.G. Cloning, molecular characterization, and chromosomal assignment of a gene encoding a second D_1 dopamine receptor subtype: differential expression pattern in rat brain compared with the D_{1A} receptor. Proc Natl Acad Sci USA. 1991; 88: 7491-7495.

9.   Sunahara, R.K., Guan, H.C., O'Dowd, B.F., Seeman, P., Laurier, L.G., Ng, G., George, S.R., Torchia, J., Van Tol, H.H., Niznik, H.B. Cloning of the gene for a human dopamine D_5 receptor with higher affinity for dopamine than D_1. Nature (Lond). 1991; 350: 614-619.

10.   Weinshank, R.L., Adham, N., Macchi, M., Olsen, M.A., Branchek, T.A., Hartig, P.R. Molecular cloning and characterization of a high affinity dopamine receptor (D_{1B}) and its pseudogene. J Biol Chem. 1991; 266: 22427-22435.

11.   Bunzow, J.R., Van Tol, H.H.M., Grandy, D.K., Albert, P., Salon, J., Christie, M.,

Machida, C.A., Neve, K.A., Civelli, O. Cloning and expression of a rat D_2 dopamine receptor cDNA. Nature (Lond). 1988; 336: 783-787.

12.   Monsma, F.J.Jr., McVittie, L.D., Gerfen, C.R., Mahan, L.C., Sibley, D.R. Multiple D_2 dopamine receptors produced by alternative RNA splicing. Nature (Lond). 1989; 342: 926-929.

13.   Sokoloff, P., Giros, B., Martres, MP., Bouthenet, M.L., Schwartz, J.C. Molecular cloning and characterization of a novel dopamine receptor (D_3) as a target for neuroleptics. Nature (Lond). 1990; 347: 146-151.

14.   Van Tol, H.H.M., Bunzow, J.R., Guan, H.C., Sunahara, R.K., Seeman, P., Niznik, H.B., Civelli, O. Cloning of the gene for a human dopamine D_4 receptor with high affinity for the antipsychotic clozapine. Nature (Lond). 1991; 350: 610-614.

15.   Bouvier, C., VanTol, H.H.M., Bunzow, J., Johnson, R.A., Niznik, H., Civelli, O. Cloning and functional characterization of the dopamine D_4 receptor. Soc Neurosci Abs. 1991; 17: 598.

16.   Falardeau, P., Godinot, N., Giros, B., Schwartz, J.C., Caron, M.G. Coupling of the rat D3 dopamine receptor to adenylyl cyclase in GH4C1 cells. Soc Neurosci Abs. 1991; 17: 356.

17.   Vallar, L., Muca, C., Magni, M., Albert, P., Bunzou, J., Meldolesi, J., Civelli, O. Differential coupling of dopaminergic D2 receptors expressed in different cell types. J Biol Chem. 1990; 265: 10320-10326.

18.   Minowa, M.T., Minowa, T., Monsma, F.J.Jr., Sibley, D.R., Mouradian, M.M. Characterization of the 5' flanking region of the human D_{1A} dopamine receptor gene. Proc Natl Acad Sci USA . 1992; 89: 3045-3049.

19.   Sibley, D.R., Monsma, F.J.Jr. Molecular biology of dopamine receptors. Trends Pharmacol Sci. 1992; 13: 61-69.

20.   Jose, P.A., Raymond, J.R., Bates, M.D., Aperia, A., Felder, R.A., Carey, R.M. The renal dopamine receptors. J Am Soc Nephrol. 1992; 2: 1265-1278.

21.   Andersen, P.H., Gingrich, J.A., Bates, M.D., Dearry, A., Falardeau, P., Senogles, S.E., Caron, M.G.. Dopamine receptor subtypes: beyond the D_1/D_2 classification. Trends Pharmacol Sci. 1990; 11: 231-236.

22.   Aperia, A., Meister, B., Hokfelt, T. Dopamine: An intrarenal hormone. Contemp Issues Nephrol. 1991; 23: 315-338.

23.   Lokhandwala, M. F., Amenta, F. Anatomical distribution and function of dopamine

receptors in the kidney. FASEB J. 1991; 5: 3023-3030.

24. Lacey, M.G., Mercuri, N.B., North, R.A. Dopamine acts on D_2 receptors to increase potassium conductance in neurones of the rat substantia nigra zona compacta. J Physiol. 1987; 398: 397-416.

25. Felder, C.C., Blecher, M., Jose, P.A.: Dopamine-1 mediated stimulation of phospholipase C activity in rat renal cortical membranes. J Biol Chem. 1989; 264: 8739-8745.

26. Felder, C.C., Jose, P.A., Axelrod, J. The dopamine-1 agonist, SKF 82526, stimulates phospholipase-C activity independent of adenylate cyclase. J Pharmacol Exp Ther. 1989; 248: 171-175.

27. Vyas, S.J., Jadhav, A.L., Eichberg, J., Lokhandwala, M.F. Dopamine receptor-mediated activation of phospholipase C is associated with natriuresis during high salt intake. Am J Physiol. 1992; 62: F494-F498.

28. Mahan, L.C., Burch, R.M., Monsma, F.J.Jr., Sibley, D.R. Expression of striatal D_1 dopamine receptors coupled to inositol phosphate production and Ca^{2+} mobilization in *Xenopus* oocytes. Proc Natl Acad Sci. 1990; 87: 2196-2200.

29. Rodrigues, P.D.S., Dowling, J.E. Dopamine induces neurite retraction in horizontal cells via diacylglycerol and protein kinase C. Proc Natl Acad Sci USA. 1990; 87: 9693-9697.

30. Monsma, F.J. Jr., Shen, Y., Mahan, L.C., Sibley, D.R. Identification of a novel G protein-coupled receptor which exhibits high homology to cloned dopamine receptors. FASEB J. 1992; 6: A15569#3591.

31. Strader, C.D., Candelore, M.R., Hill, W.S., Sigal, I.S., Dixon, R.A. Identification of two serine residues involved in agonist activation of the β-adrenergic receptor. J Biol Chem. 1989; 264: 13572-13578.

32. Neve, K.A., Henningsen, R.A., Spanoyannis, A., Neve, R.L. Pivotal role for aspartate-80 in the regulation of dopamine D_2 receptor affinity for drugs and inhibition of adenylyl cyclase. Mol Pharmacol. 1991; 39: 733-739.

33. Pollock, N.J., Manelli, A.M., Hutchins, C.W., MacKenzie, R.G., Frail, D.E. Ligand binding domains of the human D1 receptor determined by single site mutations. Soc Neurosci Abs. 1991; 17: 85 #36.8

34. Giros, B., Martres, M.P., Pilon, P., Sokoloff, P., Schwartz, J.C.. Shorter variants of the D_3 dopamine receptor produced through various patterns of alternative splicing. Biochem Biophys Res Comm 1991; 175: 1584-1591.

35.   Todd, R.D., Khurana, T.S., Sajovic, P., Stone, K.R., O'Malley, K.L. Cloning of
       ligand-specific cell lines via gene transfer: identification of a D2 dopamine receptor
       subtype. Proc Natl Acad Sci USA. 1989; 86: 10134-10138.

36.   Piomelli, D, Pilon, C., Giros, B., Sokoloff, P., Martres, M.P., Schwartz, J.C.
       Dopamine activation of the arachidonic acid cascade as a basis for D_1/D_2 receptor
       synergism. Nature (Lond). 1991; 353: 164-167.

37.   Felder, C. C., Williams, H. L. , Axelrod, J. L.. A transduction pathway associated
       with receptors coupled to the inhibitory guanine nucleotide binding protein G_i that
       amplifies ATP-mediated arachidonic acid release. Proc. Natl. Acad. Sci. USA. 1991;
       88: 6477-6480,

38.   Goldberg, L.I., Kohli, J.D., Glock, D. Conclusive evidence for two subtypes of
       peripheral dopamine receptors. In:Woodruff GN, Poat JA, Roberts PJ, eds.
       Dopaminergic Systems and Their Regulation. Macmillan, London, 1986: 195-212.

39.   Sidhu, A., Vachvanichsanong, P., Jose, P.A., Felder, R.A. Persistent defective
       coupling of dopamine-1 receptors to G proteins after solubilization from kidney
       proximal tubules of hypertensive rats. J Clin Invest. 1992; 89: 789-793.

40.   Kinoshita, S., Ohlstein, S.E.H., Felder, R.A. Dopamine-1 receptors in rat proximal
       convoluted tubule: regulation by intrarenal dopamine. Am J Physiol. 1990; 258:
       F1068-F1074.

41.   Felder, C.C., McKelvey, A.M, Gitler, M.S., Eisner, G.M., Jose PA. Dopamine
       receptor subtypes in renal brush border and basolateral membranes. Kidney Int.
       1989; 36: 183-193.

42.   Felder, R.A., Blecher, M., Calcagno, P.L., Jose, P.A. Dopamine receptors
       in the proximal tubule of the rabbit. Am J Physiol. 1984; 247: F499-F505.

43.   Felder, R.A., Blecher, M., Eisner, G.M., Jose, P.A. Cortical tubular and
       glomerular dopamine receptors in the rat kidney. Am JPhysiol. 1984; 246: F557-
       F568.

44.   Meister, B., Fryckstedt, J., Schalling, M., Cortes, R., Hokfelt, T., Aperia, A.,
       Hemmings, H.C. Jr., Nairn, A.C., Ehrlich, M., Greengard, P. Dopamine- and
       cAMP-regulated phosphoprotein (DARPP-32) and dopamine DA_1 agonist-sensitive
       Na^+,K^+-ATPase in renal tubule cells. Proc Natl Acad Sci USA. 1989; 86: 8068-
       8072.

45.   Ohbu, K., Felder, R.A. Dopamine-receptors in the cortical collecting duct. Am J
       Physiol. 1991; 261: F890-F895.

46. Satoh,T., Cohen, H.T., Katz, A.I. Intracellular signalling in the regulation of renal Na-K-ATPase. 1. Role of cyclic AMP and phospholipase A$_2$. J Clin Invest. 1992; 89: 1496-1500.

47. Takemoto, F., Satoh, T., Cohen, H.T., Katz, A.I. Localization of dopamine-l receptors along the microdissected rat nephron. Pflugers Arch. 1991; 419: 243-248.

48. Huo, T., Ye, M.Q., Healy, D.P. Characterization of dopamine receptor (DA$_{2K}$) in the kidney inner medulla. Proc Natl Acad Sci USA. 1991; 88: 3170-3174.

49. Yamaguchi, I., Canessa, L.M., Monsma, F.J.Jr., Sibley, D.R., Mouradian, M.M., Jose, P.A., Felder, R.A. D$_{1A}$ dopamine receptor mRNA in proximal tubules of normotensive and spontaneously hypertensive rat (SHR). Pediatr Res. 1992; 31: 346A.

50. Jose, P.A., Canessa, L.M., Monsma, F.J.Jr., Sibley, D.R., Felder, R.A., Mouradian, M.M. Regional distribution of the D$_{1B}$ dopamine receptor mRNA in the kidney. Pediatr Res. 1992; 31: 336A.

51. Jose, P.A., Felder, R.A., Robillard, J.E., Albrecht, F., Sibley, D.R., Monsma, F.J.Jr., Mouradian, M.M. Renal proximal tubular dopamine-1 (D$_1$) receptor mRNA identified by ribonuclease protection assay (RPA) and relationship to renal Na$^+$/H$^+$ exchanger in normotensive and spontaneously hypertensive rat (SHR). Pediatr Res. 1991; 29: 345 A.

52. Jose, P.A., Monsma, F.J.Jr., Sibley, D.R., Mouradian, M.M., Felder, R.A. Significance of the D$_{1A}$ and D$_{1B}$ receptor mRNA in renal proximal tubules in Wistar Kyoto (WKY) and spontaneously hypertensive rat (SHR). Am J Hypertens. 1992; 5: 6A.

53. Meister, B., Holgert, H., Aperia, A., and Hokfelt T. Dopamine D1 receptor m RNA in rat kidney. localization by in situ hybridization. Acta Physiol. Scand. 1991;143:447-449.

54. Monsma, F.J.Jr., Shen, Y., Gerfen, C.R., Mahan, L.C., Jose, P.A., Mouradian, M.M., Sibley, D.R. Molecular cloning of a novel D$_1$ dopamine receptor from rat kidney. Soc Neurosci Abs. 1991; 17: 85.

55. O'Malley, K.L., Harmon, S., Tang, L., Han, S., Todd, R.D. The rat dopamine D4 receptor: sequence, gene structure, and demonstration of expression in the cardiovascular system. New Biol. 1992; 4: 137-146.

Pharmacological Studies of Dopamine Receptors in Cultured Renal Epithelial Cells

D.P. Healy, T. Huo, V. Bogdanov and
A. Grenader

Department of Pharmacology, The Mount Sinai School of Medicine,
New York, NY 10029, USA

ABSTRACT

The pharmacological properties of dopamine receptor subtypes were examined in cultured renal epithelial cells. The porcine renal epithelial cell line, LLC-PK$_1$, was shown to express a dopamine-1 (DA$_1$) receptor coupled to stimulation of adenylyl cyclase. The DA$_1$ agonist A68930 was a potent full agonist in LLC-PK$_1$ cells, whereas SK&F 82526, SK&F 85174 and (+)6-Br-APB were only partial agonists. Inner medullary collecting duct (IMCD) cells were shown to bind ^{3}H-spiperone or ^{3}H-domperidone with a similar pharmacological profile as the striatal and pituitary D$_2$ receptors, but with lower affinity. Northern blot analysis of kidney inner medulla mRNA with a D$_2$ receptor cDNA was negative. Photoaffinity cross linking, however, with N-(p-azido-m-[^{125}I]iodophenethyl)spiperone resulted in labeling of similar size proteins (M$_r \approx$120,000) from striatum, pituitary and inner medulla. DA stimulated PGE$_2$ production in cultured IMCD cells, an effect that could be blocked by DA$_2$ antagonists or pertussis toxin. Thus, IMCD cells appear to express a novel G protein-coupled DA$_2$-like receptor, which we have termed DA$_{2K}$. These results further suggest that pharmacological and physiological studies with cultured renal epithelial cells may provide new insights into renal dopamine receptor mechanisms.

INTRODUCTION

Exogenously administered dopamine (DA) elicits natriuretic and diuretic responses in a variety of species (1). These effects can be blocked by DA antagonists (2). Both dopamine-1 (DA$_1$) and DA$_2$ receptors have been characterized in the kidney (2-4). The DA$_1$ receptor is localized primarily in proximal tubules (3) and the DA$_2$ receptor primarily in the inner medullary collecting ducts (4). The effects of exogenously administered DA appear to be mediated primarily by DA$_1$ receptors (2), but recent studies indicate that DA$_2$ receptors in the inner medulla may also be involved in mediating responses to DA (5,6).

The renal DA_1 receptor has been characterized in homogenate preparations and microdissected tubules. DA has been reported to increase adenylyl cyclase activity (2) and phosphoinositide turnover (7,8), although the latter effects appear to require higher doses of DA. DA has been reported to inhibit Na-K-ATPase activity in proximal tubules and Na-H antiporter activity in brush border membrane vesicles (9,10). These results suggest that DA may elicit natriuresis by inhibition of sodium reabsorption through a direct action on tubular DA receptors.

An alternative approach for study of DA receptor mechanisms is to use cultured renal epithelial cells. The porcine renal epithelial cell line, $LLC\text{-}PK_1$, has been used extensively to study of proximal tubule cell function. In addition, we have shown that inner medullary collecting ducts express a DA_2-like receptor that we have termed DA_{2K} (4). This report will summarize the principal findings of studies that examined DA_1 receptor mechanisms in $LLC\text{-}PK_1$ cells and DA_{2K} receptor mechanisms in IMCD cells.

LLC-PK₁ cell DA₁ receptors

At confluency $LLC\text{-}PK_1$ cells form a polarized monolayer and express transport properties consistent with a proximal tubule cell phenotype (11). Microdissected proximal tubules have been shown to increase adenylyl cyclase activity in response to DA_1 agonist stimulation (12). $LLC\text{-}PK_1$ cells were tested for the presence of a functional DA_1 receptor by measuring cAMP accumulation in response to DA stimulation. DA increased cAMP accumulation in $LLC\text{-}PK_1$ cells with an EC_{50} of 1.5 μM and an E_{max} approximately 8-10 fold above basal levels (13). This effect was blocked by the DA_1 antagonists SK&F 83566 and SCH 23390 but not by DA_2 or β-adrenergic antagonists. Stimulation of cAMP accumulation was not seen in the absence of the phosphodiesterase inhibitor isobutylmethyl-xanthine, indicating that the DA-mediated increase in cAMP accumulation was due to stimulation of adenylyl cyclase and not inhibition of phosphodiesterase. Interestingly, L-dopa also increased cAMP accumulation in $LLC\text{-}PK_1$ cells (13). This effect was blocked by carbidopa, an inhibitor of aromatic L-amino acid decarboxylase. The response to L-dopa is consistent with evidence that $LLC\text{-}PK_1$ cells contain high levels of aromatic L-amino acid decarboxylase, produce DA from

L-dopa, and secrete DA across the apical membrane (13). Moreover, these results suggest that locally produced DA can act as a paracrine substance to stimulate apical membrane DA_1 receptors that are coupled to adenylyl cyclase (13).

The pharmacology of the LLC-PK_1 cell DA_1 receptor was further examined by comparing the ability of various DA_1 agonists to stimulate cAMP accumulation. Fenoldopam has been widely used as an DA_1-selective agonist and has been proposed as a possible therapeutic agent for treatment of hypertension and congestive heart failure (14). However, although fenoldopam was highly potent, it was only a partial agonist at DA_1 receptors in LLC-PK_1 cells (intrinsic activity 37% of DA) (15). Indeed, the partial agonist properties of fenoldopam resulted in it acting as an antagonist in the presence of the full agonist DA, with a pA_2 value comparable to its EC_{50} value (15). Fenoldopam is therefore a low efficacy DA_1 agonist at DA_1 receptors in LLC-PK_1 cells. These findings suggest that fenoldopam may not be as efficacious an agent for treatment of hypertension or congestive heart failure as would a full agonist. These results led us to search for a high potency full agonist at DA_1 receptors in LLC-PK_1 cells. The mixed DA_1/DA_2 agonist SK&F 85174 and the DA_1 agonist (+)-3-allyl-6-bromo-7,8-dihyroxy-1-phenyl-2,3,4,5-tetrahydro-1H-3-benzazepin [(+)6-Br-APB] (16) were also only partial agonists in LLC-PK_1 cells (17, unpublished observations). We determined that A68930 [(1R,3S)-1-aminomethyl-5,6-dihydroxy-3-phenylisochroman, Abbott Labs, Abbott Park, IL] was a highly potent (EC_{50} 12.7 nM) full agonist at stimulating cAMP accumulation in LLC-PK_1 cells (17). The pharmacology of A68930 indicated that it was a DA_1 selective agonist (17,18). These results suggest that A68930 may be a useful agonist to study the physiological properties of renal DA_1 receptors.

Based on the results of in vitro studies with LLC-PK_1 cells, we can propose the following model for DA_1 receptors in proximal tubules (Figure 1). L-Dopa is taken up by proximal tubule cells via the sodium-amino acid co-transporter (11). L-Dopa is converted intracellularly by AADC to DA, which is then secreted across the apical surface of the cells. DA reaches concentrations within the apical membrane sufficient to activate DA_1 receptors. DA has been reported to stimulate adenylyl cyclase as well as phosphoinositide hydrolysis in proximal tubule cells (7,8,12). Therefore, the intracellular messenger secondary to DA_1 receptor activation is

represented in Figure 1 as a "black box". Likewise, the tubular response to DA
stimulation is also unresolved. DA has been shown to inhibit sodium transport in
the proximal tubules, either by inhibition of the Na-K-ATPase or the Na-H
antiporter (9,10). The precise mechanism is unknown by may involve cAMP
mediated increase in protein kinase A activity or a synergistic action with DA_2
receptors (9). Protein kinase A is known to inhibit Na-H antiporter activity (20).
The effect of DA_1 receptor stimulation on sodium transport in LLC-PK$_1$ cells is
unknown. Preliminary evidence from LLC-PK$_1$ cells indicates that DA does not
inhibit ouabain-sensitive ^{86}Rb uptake (Grenader and Healy, unpublished observations).
Further studies with the LLC-PK$_1$ cells in vitro may provide insights as to the
mechanism of DA-mediated inhibition of sodium transport by the proximal tubules.

Inner medullary collecting duct DA_{2K} receptors

Radioligand binding studies had indicated that DA_2 receptors are present in
kidney (4) but their role in mediation of the effects of exogenously applied DA
remains unclear. The general belief was that DA_2 receptors are present on
sympathetic nerve terminals and modulated the release of norepinephrine. We
sought to determine the localization of renal DA_2 receptors by autoradiography with
^{3}H-spiperone, a DA_2-selective antagonist. ^{3}H-Spiperone binding sites were diffusely
distributed within the cortex but highly concentrated on inner medullary collecting
ducts (4). ^{3}H-Spiperone binding was saturable with a K_d of 17 nM and a B_{max} of
935 fmol/mg protein (4). The pharmacological profile of the ^{3}H-spiperone binding,
however, was somewhat different from that seen in the striatum or pituitary, tissues
known to express the D_2 receptor. In general, the rank order profile was similar to
that seen in brain or pituitary, but the affinities were shifted to lower values.
Similar results were seen using ^{3}H-domperidone, a DA_2-selective antagonist, and
cultured inner medullary collecting duct (IMCD) cells (21). These results led us to
determine whether the size of the protein being labeled in the kidney was similar to
that seen in brain and pituitary. Photoaffinity cross-linking with N-(*p*-azido-*m*-
[^{125}I]iodophenethyl)spiperone yielded labeling of protein of $M_r{\approx}120,000$ in striatum,
pituitary and kidney medulla (4), suggesting that the IMCD ^{3}H-spiperone and ^{3}H-
domperidone binding site was similar to the DA_2 receptor. Interestingly, Northern
blot hybridization with a brain D_2 receptor cDNA and kidney inner medulla RNA

was negative (4), strongly suggesting that the inner medulla site was not identical to the brain/pituitary D_2 receptor. Thus the molecular identity of the IMCD DA receptor is still unknown, but the present findings suggest that it is DA_2-like. We have tentatively termed this site DA_{2K} (4,21).

Further studies were conducted to determine whether the DA_{2K} site in IMCD cells represents a functional receptor. Initial studies with cultured IMCD cells indicated that DA_2 agonist stimulation did not inhibit adenylyl cyclase activity. The precise localization of the ^3H-spiperone binding sites to the inner medulla led us to examine other possibilities. Prostaglandin E_2 (PGE_2) is the major eicosanoid in rat kidney and is known to be produced primarily in the inner medulla (22). DA has been reported to increase PGE_2 levels in the urine (23). We determined that DA produced a dose-dependent increase in PGE_2 production, with an EC_{50} of 11 μM and an E_{max} of 2.3 fold higher than basal (4-6). This response was blocked by DA_2 antagonists (4-6). We then tested a variety of inhibitors to determine the mechanism of the DA-mediated PGE_2 production (5). Indomethacin (10 μM), a cyclooxygenase inhibitor, suppressed PGE_2 synthesis to less than 5% of basal levels and completely blocked the DA response, verifying that PGE_2 was being produced enzymatically through the cyclooxygenase pathway. Nordihydroguaiaretic acid, a lipoxygenase inhibitor, had no effect on DA-stimulated PGE_2 production. Quinacrine, a phospholipase A_2 inhibitor, inhibited DA-stimulated PGE_2 synthesis, suggesting that the major source of arachidonic acid was through hydrolysis of membrane phospholipids by PLA_2. 8-(Diethylamino)octyl-3,4,5-trimethoxybenzoate hydrochloride, an intracellular calcium blocker, also suppressed DA-stimulated PGE_2 synthesis. In contrast, the voltage-dependent calcium channel blockers, verapamil and diltiazem (100 μM), had no effect. Neomycin, an inhibitor of polyphosphatidylinositol hydrolysis by phospholipase C, did not inhibit DA-stimulated PGE_2 levels. The phorbol ester tetradecanoyl phorbol acetate (TPA), a stimulator of the calcium/phospholipid-dependent protein kinase, protein kinase C (PK-C), increased basal PGE_2 levels almost 10 fold. The PK-C inhibitor, 1-(5-isoquinolinylsulfonyl)-2-methylpiperazine (H-7), at doses that blocked the TPA-stimulated response, failed to block DA-stimulated PGE_2 production in IMCD cells. These results suggest that PK-C was probably not involved in the DA-stimulated increase in PGE_2. Finally, DA receptors are known to couple to their effector

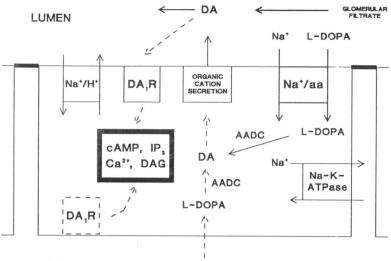

FIG. 1   Model for DA$_1$ receptor mechanisms in a proximal tubule cell.   Solid
lines represent processes shown to exist in proximal tubule and/or LLC-PK$_1$ cells.
Dashed lines represent processes that are speculative.   The intracellular secondary
messenger system is represented as a black box.   See text for details.
Abbreviations: DA$_1$R, dopamine-1 receptor; AADC, aromatic L-amino acid
decarboxylase; Na$^+$/aa, sodium-amino acid co-transporter; Na$^+$/H$^+$, sodium-hydrogen
antiporter; IP$_3$, inositol triphosphate; DAG, diacylglycerol.

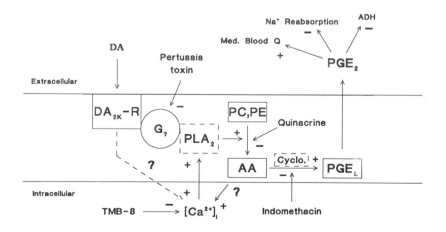

FIG. 2   Model for DA$_{2K}$ receptor mechanisms in an inner medullary collecting
duct cell.   See text for details.   Abbreviations: AA, arachidonic acid; PLA$_2$,
phospholipase A$_2$; PC, phosphatidylcholine; PE, phosphatidylethanolamine; cyclo,
cyclooxygenase; TMB-8, 8-(Diehtylamino)octyl-3,4,5-trimethoxybenzoate; med. blood
Q, medullary blood flow; ADH, antidiuretic hormone.

proteins via guanine nucleotide binding proteins (G proteins). Pertussis toxin (PT) catalyzes the ADP-ribosylation of some G proteins, reducing their ability to couple to effector proteins. We tested whether the DA-stimulated PGE_2 response was sensitive to PT treatment. PT (100 ng/ml) completely abolished the DA-stimulated PGE_2 production, indicating that the DA_{2K} receptor-mediated response was dependent on coupling to a PT-sensitive G protein. PT had no effect on arachidonic acid (10 μM) stimulation of PGE_2 formation, indicating that the PT was interfering with events proximal to cyclooxygenase, presumably at the level of the receptor-G protein interaction (5).

These results suggest the following model for DA-stimulation of PGE_2 production in IMCD cells (Figure 2). DA binds to DA_{2K} receptors coupled to PLA_2 via a pertussis toxin-sensitive G protein. Activation of PLA_2 stimulates breakdown of phosphatidylcholine or phosphatidylethanolamine to generate arachidonic acid which enters the cyclooxygenase pathway leading to generation of PGE_2. The demonstration that DA-stimulated PGE_2 production requires intracellular calcium suggests that additional mechanisms that result in release of calcium from intracellular stores may also be involved. The stimulation PGE_2 production by IMCD cells by DA may be physiologically significant with regards to DA action in the kidney. PGE_2 is the major eicosanoid formed by the kidney, with the highest levels being produced in the inner medulla (22). PGE_2 influences water and electrolyte movement across outer medullary collecting duct and IMCD by both direct and indirect processes (24). Direct effects of PGE_2 on collecting ducts include inhibition of sodium transport (24), possibly by inhibition of Na^+-K^+-ATPase activity (25), and inhibition of urea reabsorption (24). Indirect effects of PGE_2 on the collecting ducts include increases in medullary blood flow and reduction in inner medullary interstitial pressure, thereby diminishing the osmotic driving force for water reabsorption across the collecting ducts (24), and inhibition of vasopressin-stimulated increases in collecting duct water permeability (22). Thus the stimulation of PGE_2 production by DA is consistent with the known effects of DA on whole kidney physiology. Furthermore, these results suggest that activation of DA receptors in the inner medulla may contribute to the natriuretic/diuretic effects of DA on the kidney.

D.P. Healy *et al.*

In summary, these studies indicate that the proximal tubule-like renal epithelial LLC-PK$_1$ cell line and primary cultures of IMCD cells are useful models to study DA$_1$ and DA$_{2K}$ receptor mechanisms in vitro. Further characterization of the pharmacological, physiological and molecular properties of tubular DA receptors should provide insights into the role of tubular DA receptors in mediating the natriuretic effects of DA on the kidney.

REFERENCES

1. Goldberg, L.I. Cardiovascular and renal actions of dopamine: potential clinical applications. Pharmacol Rev. 1972; 24: 1-29.

2. Felder, R.A., Felder, C.C., Eisner, G.M., Jose, P.A. The dopamine receptor in adult and maturing kidney. Am J Physiol. 1989; 257: F315-F327.

3. Huo, T., Healy, D.P. Autoradiographic localization of dopamine DA$_1$ receptors in rat kidney with [^{3}H]Sch 23390. Am J Physiol. 1989; 257: F414-F423.

4. Huo, T., Ye, M.Q., Healy, D.P. Characterization of a dopamine receptor (DA$_{2K}$) in the kidney inner medulla. Proc Nat Acad Sci. 1991; 88: 3170-3174.

5. Huo, T., Healy, D.P. Prostaglandin E$_2$ production in IMCD cells. I. Stimulation by dopamine. Am J Physiol. 1991; 261: F647-F654.

6. Huo, T., Grenader, A., Blandina, P., Healy, D.P. Prostaglandin E$_2$ production in IMCD cells. II. Possible role for locally formed dopamine. Am J Physiol. 1991; 261: F655-F662.

7. Felder, C.C., Blecher, M., Jose, P.A. Dopamine-1 receptor-mediated stimulation of phospholipase C activity in rat renal cortical membranes. J Biol Chem. 1989; 264: 8739-8745.

8. Vyas, S.J., Eichberg, J., Lokhandwala, M.F. Characterization of receptors involved in dopamine-induced activation of phospholipase-C in rat renal cortex. J Pharmacol Exp Ther. 1992; 260: 143-139.

9. Aperia, A., Bertorello, A., Seri, I. Dopamine causes inhibition of Na$^+$-K$^+$-ATPase activity in rat proximal convoluted tubule segments. Am J Physiol. 1987; 252: F39-F45.

10. Felder, C.C., Cambell, T., Albrecht, F., Jose, P.A. Dopamine inhibits Na$^+$-H$^+$ exchanger activity in renal BBMV by stimulation of adenylate cyclase. Am J Physiol. 1990; 259: F297-F303.

11. Rabito, C.A. Sodium co-transport processes in renal epithelial cell lines.

Mineral Electrolye Metab. 1986; 12: 32-41.

12.   Kinoshita, S., Ohlstein, E.H., Felder, R.A.   Dopamine-1 receptors in rat proximal convoluted tubule: regulation by intrarenal dopamine.   Am J Physiol. 1990; 258: F1068-F1074.

13.   Grenader, A., Healy, D.P.   Locally formed dopamine stimulates cAMP accumulation in LLC-PK$_1$ cells via a DA$_1$ receptor.   Am J Physiol. 1991; 260: F906-F912.

14.   Holcslaw, T.L., Beck, T.R.   Clinical experience with intravenous fenoldopam.   Am J Hyperten. 1990; 3: 120S-125S.

15.   Grenader, A., Healy, D.P.   Fenoldopam is a partial agonist at dopamine-1 (DA$_1$) receptors in LLC-PK$_1$ Cells.   J Pharmacol Exp Ther. 1991; 258: 193-198.

16.   Neumeyer, J.L., Baindur, N., Niznik, H.B., Guan, H.C., Seeman, P.   (±)-3-Allyl-6-bromo-7,8-dihydroxy-1-phenyl-2,3,4,5-tetrahydro-1H-3-benzazepin,   a new high-affinity D1 dopamine receptor ligand: synthesis and structure-activity relationship.   J Med Chem. 1991; 34: 3366-3371.

17.   Grenader, A., Healy, D.P.   A68930 is a potent, full agonist at dopamine-1 (DA$_1$) receptors in renal epithelial LLC-PK$_1$ cells.   Br J Pharmacol. 1992; 106: 229-230.

18.   DeNinno, M.P., Schoenleber, R., MacKenzie, R., Britton, D.R., Asin, K.E., Briggs, C., Trugman, J.M., Ackerman, M., Artman, L., Bednarz, L., Bhatt, R., Curzon, P., Gomez, E., Kang, C.H., Stittsworth, J., Kebabian, J.W.   A68930: a potent agonist selective for the dopamine D$_1$ receptor.   Eur J Pharmacol. 1991; 199: 209-219.

19.   Baines, A.D., Chan, W.   Production of urine free dopamine from DOPA; a micropuncture study.   Life Sci. 1980; 26: 253-259.

20.   Weinman, E.J., Dubinsky, W., Shenolikar, S.   Regulation of the renal Na+-H+ exchanger by protein phosphorylation.   Kidney Int. 1989; 36: 519-525.

21.   Huo, T., Healy, D.P. ^{3}H-Domperidone binding to the kidney inner medullary collecting duct dopamine-2K (DA$_{2K}$) receptor.   J Pharmacol Exp Ther. 1991; 258: 424-428.

22.   Dunn, M. J.   Hormones and Autacoids produced in the kidney.   In: Renal Endocrinology.   M. J. Dunn (ed.).   Baltimore, Maryland, Williams and Wilkins, 1983, p. 1-74.

23.   Yoshimura, M., Takashina, R., Takahasi, H., Ijichi, H.   Role of renal nerves and dopamine on prostaglandin E release from the kidney of rats.   Agents and Actions 1987; 22: 93-99.

24.   Stokes, J. B.   Integrated actions of renal medullary prostaglandins in the

control of water excretion. Am J Physiol 1981; 240: F471-F480.

25.   Jabs, K., Zeidel, M.L., Silva, P.   Prostaglandin E_2 inhibits Na^+-K^+-ATPase activity in the inner medullary collecting duct. Am J Physiol. 257: F424-F430.

ACKNOWLEDGMENTS

We would like to thank Dr. John Kebabian (Research Biochemicals Inc., Natick, MA) for supplying (+)6-Br-APB and Dr. J. Paul Hieble (SmithKline Beecham, Pharmaceuticals, King of Prussia, PA) for supplying SF&F 85174 and SK&F 82526. This work was supported by the American Heart Association (Grant-in-Aid #91014490), the Irma T. Hirschl Foundation, and the National Institutes of Health (HL 42585).   DPH is an Established Investigator of the American Heart Association.

Signal Transduction in the Action of Dopamine in Rat Renal Tubules

Takeo Satoh, Herbert T. Cohen and
Adrian I. Katz

Department of Medicine, University of Chicago Pritzker School of
Medicine, Chicago, Illinois, IL 60637, USA

Dopamine inhibits tubular sodium reabsorption, which is attributed in part to inhibition of Na-K-ATPase in the proximal convoluted tubule (PCT) (1). This effect on the Na:K pump appears to be independent of altered sodium entry (2), although dopamine inhibits the proximal tubule Na:H exchanger as well (3,4). Pump inhibition by dopamine in the PCT requires activation of both the DA_1 and DA_2 receptor subtypes (5), and of protein kinase C (6). It was not known, however, whether dopamine inhibits Na-K-ATPase activity in other nephron segments. We therefore sought to determine whether dopamine receptors are present beyond the proximal tubule and, because the collecting duct is responsible for the fine control of sodium excretion, whether dopamine inhibits Na-K-ATPase in this part of the nephron. The present paper summarizes our recent work addressing these issues, and emphasizes studies aimed at clarifying the signaling mechanisms involved in the interaction of dopamine with the Na:K pump in the cortical collecting duct (CCD) (7-10).

The experiments described below were performed in vitro on microdissected rat renal tubules, using techniques described in detail in the studies cited. In brief, binding experiments were done on single tubule segments (average length 2 mm) incubated for 60 min at room temperature in 1 µl buffer containing the high specific radioactivity ligand ^{125}I-SCH 23982. Nonspecific binding was determined in the presence of excess unlabeled SCH 23390 (7). Na-K-ATPase activity was also measured in single pieces of tubule, by the hydrolysis of $[\gamma\text{-}^{32}P]ATP$ in the presence or absence of 4 mM ouabain (8-10). Tubules were preincubated with agonists for 15-30 min at $37^{\circ}C$ prior to the ATPase assay.

We first determined the location and density of DA_1 receptors along the microdissected rat nephron using the specific and selective DA_1 receptor ligand $^{125}I\text{-SCH}$ 23982. DA_1 receptors were most abundant in the proximal tubule, but were present in other segments as well, especially in the collecting duct, which displayed the next highest receptor concentration. Rosenthal plots of binding data from the PCT and cortical collecting duct (CCD) revealed that the DA_1 receptor affinity appeared to be higher in the latter (K_D 16.7 and 6.2 nM, respectively) (7).

The presence of ample $^{125}I\text{-SCH}$ 23982 binding sites in the CCD led us to examine whether, as in the PCT, dopamine also inhibited Na-K-ATPase activity in this segment. Indeed, dopamine inhibited CCD Na-K-ATPase in a dose-dependent manner (7), and did so to a greater extent (40-55% vs. 24%) than in PCT (8).

To determine which dopamine receptor subtype was responsible for the CCD pump inhibition, we used the DA_1 agonist fenoldopam, the highly selective DA_1 antagonist SCH 23390, and the DA_2 agonist quinpirole. Fenoldopam alone reproduced the dopamine effect on Na-K-ATPase in similar dose-dependent fashion, and its action was completely blocked by SCH 23390. In contrast, quinpirole by itself had no effect on the pump, and in combination with fenoldopam it failed to inhibit it further (8). Taken together, these findings strongly suggest that the effect of dopamine on CCD Na-K-ATPase occurs through activation of the DA_1, but not the DA_2 receptor.

Our results in the PCT differed from those in the CCD, in that fenoldopam alone did not reproduce the pump inhibition by dopamine, but required the added presence of quinpirole. Quinpirole alone, however, exerted no effect on Na-K-ATPase. Thus unlike the CCD, the results in PCT suggest that dopamine acts on both the DA_1 and DA_2 receptors to effect pump inhibition, a finding that confirms earlier studies by others in this nephron segment (5). From the above evidence we concluded that the natriuretic action of dopamine likely occurs at both proximal and distal sites, and that this effect is due, at least in part, to inhibition of Na-K-ATPase, albeit by different mechanisms in these two regions of the nephron.

Because activation of the DA_1 receptor is linked to adenylyl cyclase, to evaluate the mechanism of the dopamine-induced pump inhibition in the CCD we began by measuring cAMP accumulation in response to dopamine-receptor agonists and antagonists in this segment (8) with a sensitive radioimmunoassay (11). Dopamine caused a two-fold increase in cAMP accumulation, an effect reproduced by fenoldopam alone and blocked by the addition of SCH 23390, whereas quinpirole alone did not alter cAMP content (8). These results provide further evidence that in the CCD dopamine exerts its effects via DA_1 receptors, and suggest that DA_1 receptor-mediated increases in cAMP may be the principal effector mechanism involved in CCD pump inhibition.

Cyclic AMP agonists have been shown to inhibit Na:K pump activity in nonrenal tissues (12,13), and dibutyryl cAMP has the same action in rat medullary thick ascending limbs (14). To confirm the role of cAMP in CCD we demonstrated next that other agents that increase cell cAMP by different mechanisms (arginine vasopressin [AVP], forskolin [which stimulates adenylyl cyclase activity directly], and dibutyryl cAMP), like the DA_1 agonist fenoldopam, also inhibit the pump in CCD, and do so to a comparable extent (9). The inhibitory effect of dopamine and fenoldopam was then shown to be mediated via the cAMP-dependent protein kinase (PKA) pathway, as it was completely blocked by both the adenylyl cyclase inhibitor 2',5'-dideoxyadenosine and by the 20-amino acid peptide (IP_{20}) inhibitor of PKA (9). These results differ from observations in the PCT, where dopamine-induced pump inhibition was dependent on activation of protein kinase C (6), and raise the possibility that in addition to activating different receptor subtypes, dopamine acts through different cellular mechanisms in these two segments.

In our effort to further elucidate the mechanism of dopamine-induced Na-K-ATPase inhibition in the CCD, we took note of reports of eicosanoids inhibiting sodium transport, and of such effects involving cAMP (15,16). We thus postulated that the mechanism of dopamine- or cAMP-induced pump inhibition observed by us in CCD might include eicosanoid mediators. This hypothesis was confirmed in experiments in which mepacrine, an inhibitor of phospholipase A_2, completely blocked the pump inhibition by dopamine, fenoldopam, and other cAMP agonists in CCD. Further supporting a signaling role for eicosanoids, arachidonic acid inhibited the CCD pump in a dose-dependent manner, and to an extent comparable to that of dopamine (9).

A mechanism whereby PKA activates PLA_2, first proposed by Hirata (17), involves a 40-kD phospholipase inhibitory protein (lipomodulin) that loses its ability to inhibit PLA_2 activity when phosphorylated by PKA. In nonrenal tissues lipomodulin synthesis is increased by glucocorticoids (17,18), and we noted that dopamine or fenoldopam no longer inhibited the CCD pump after the tubules were preincubated with corticosterone, which suggests that lipomodulin acts between PKA and PLA_2 in dopamine- and cAMP-mediated pump inhibition in the CCD (9).

Arachidonic acid is metabolized by three main pathways, mediated by cytochrome P450-dependent monooxygenase, cyclooxygenase, and lipoxygenase, respectively. We therefore attempted to determine the role of eicosanoid products in mediating the pump inhibition by dopamine and other cAMP agonists by assessing the effect of inhibiting separately each of these pathways, as well as that of representative metabolites of each on the CCD pump (10). Inhibitors of the cytochrome P450 monooxygenase system (ethoxyresorufin or SKF 525A, both at 10^{-7} M) completely blocked the pump inhibition by dopamine and the cAMP agonists. Pretreating rats with $CoCl_2$, which depletes cytochrome P450, had similar effects. Furthermore, 12(R)-HETE, a representative product of this pathway, inhibited the pump in dose-dependent fashion. These results strongly suggest that dopamine and other cAMP agonists inhibit CCD Na-K-ATPase by activating the cytochrome P450 monooxygenase pathway of arachidonic acid metabolism (10).

Results using cyclooxygenase inhibitors indomethacin and meclofenamate were also positive, but not identical. In dose-response studies of these agents' effects on the pump inhibition by fenoldopam, 10^{-6} M indomethacin was required for near complete reversal of the fenoldopam effect, whereas meclofenamate, even at higher concentration (10^{-5} M), did not fully block the pump inhibition by this agent. [Indomethacin has been reported to inhibit monooxygenase as well, but at a higher concentration than that required for cyclooxygenase inhibition (19)]. PGE_2, a cyclooxygenase product found in the CCD (20), inhibited the Na:K pump activity in a dose-dependent manner (10) (see below). These findings suggest that the cyclooxygenase pathway may also participate in DA_1-receptor mediated pump inhibition, but that it likely plays a lesser role than the P450 system.

In contrast to the monooxygenase and cyclooxygenase branches of the arachidonic acid cascade, the lipoxygenase pathway does not participate in fenoldopam-induced pump inhibition. The lipoxygenase inhibitors nordihydroguaiaretic acid (NDGA) and A63162 failed to block the effect of fenoldopam and cAMP agonists, and leukotrienes LTB_4 or LTD_4, two key products of this pathway, did not inhibit the pump (10).

Another direction of these studies on the mechanism of dopamine- and cAMP-induced pump inhibition in the CCD was to determine whether these agents might interact directly with the pump, or in secondary fashion, e.g., by inhibiting luminal sodium entry. These experiments shed some light on the different mechanisms by which the monooxygenase and cyclooxygenase pathways operate in inhibiting Na-K-ATPase. By perfusing kidneys with a collagenase solution containing agarose, which gels upon cooling and remains permeable to water and solutes (21), we were able to obtain CCD segments with patent lumina. Sodium entry was altered using the sodium channel blocker amiloride, at a concentration (10^{-4} M) that blocks both the sodium channel and the Na:H exchanger but does not affect the Na:K pump (22), or the sodium ionophore nystatin (50 μg/ml), which makes the cells permeable to sodium so that it is no longer rate-limiting for the pump. In other experiments we eliminated Na altogether by replacing medium NaCl with choline Cl. Dopamine and fenoldopam (as well as the other cAMP agonists) inhibited the pump in these conditions of altered sodium entry just as they did in their absence, suggesting that the cAMP agonists affect the pump activity in the CCD directly, as has been proposed to be the case in the PCT (4).

12(R)-HETE and PGE_2, representative products of the cytochrome P450-monooxygenase and cyclooxygenase pathways, respectively, were used in similar experiments. 12(R)-HETE, like dopamine and fenoldopam, inhibited Na-K-ATPase under conditions of altered sodium entry, whereas PGE_2 did not (10). Such findings support the thesis that the monooxygenase pathway likely mediates the direct DA_1-induced pump inhibition and that the cyclooxygenase pathway may contribute to this effect by limiting luminal entry of sodium.

CONCLUSIONS

In addition to the proximal convoluted tubule, DA_1 receptors were detected in the cortical collecting duct, where they were found to mediate the inhibition of Na-K-ATPase by dopamine. DA_1-induced pump inhibition was found to involve activation of the cAMP-protein kinase A pathway, and subsequently stimulation of phospholipase A_2 and arachidonic acid release. The activation of PLA_2 by PKA may involve phosphorylation and deactivation of the PLA_2-inhibitor lipomodulin. In the CCD the cytochrome P450-monooxygenase pathway of the arachidonate cascade plays a major role in the modulation of Na:K pump activity by this mechanism, whereas products of the cyclooxygenase pathway may contribute to pump inhibition indirectly, by decreasing intracellular sodium availability. The events responsible for dopamine-induced pump inhibition in the PCT are currently under investigation in our laboratory.

ACKNOWLEDGMENTS

These studies were supported by grants 881092 from the American Heart Association-National Center and by a National Kidney Foundation fellowship and National Kidney Foundation of Illinois grant-in-aid to H.T.C.

REFERENCES

1. Aperia, A., Bertorello, A., Seri, I. Dopamine causes inhibition of Na^+-K^+-ATPase activity in rat proximal convoluted tubule segments. Am J Physiol. 1987; 252: F39-F45.

2. Seri, I., Kone, B.C., Gullans, S.R., Aperia, A., Brenner, B.M., Ballerman, B.J. Locally formed dopamine inhibits Na^+-K^+-ATPase activity in rat renal cortical tubule cells. Am J Physiol. 1988; 255: F666-F673.

3. Felder, C.C., Campbell, T., Albrecht, F., Jose, P.A. Dopamine inhibits Na^+-H^+ exchanger activity in renal BBMV by stimulation of adenylate cyclase. Am J Physiol. 1990; 259: F297-F303.

4. Gesek, F.A., Schoolwerth, A.C. Hormonal interactions with the proximal Na^+-H^+ exchanger. Am J Physiol. 1990; 258: F514-F521.

5. Bertorello, A., Aperia, A. Both DA_1 and DA_2 receptor agonists are necessary to inhibit NaKATPase activity in proximal tubules from rat kidney. Acta Physiol Scand. 1988; 132: 441-443.

6. Bertorello, A., Aperia, A. Na^+-K^+-ATPase is an effector protein for protein kinase C in renal proximal tubule cells. Am J Physiol. 1989; 256: F370-F373.

7. Takemoto, F., Satoh, T., Cohen, H.T., Katz, A.I. Localization of dopamine-1 receptors along the microdissected rat nephron. Pflügers Arch. 1991; 419: 243-248.

8. Takemoto, F., Cohen, H.T., Satoh, T., Katz, A.I. Dopamine inhibits Na-K-ATPase in single tubules and cultured cells from distal nephron. Pflügers Arch. 1992; (in press).

9. Satoh, T., Cohen, H.T., Katz, A.I. Intracellular signaling in the regulation of renal Na-K-ATPase: I. Role of cyclic AMP and phospholipase A_2. J Clin Invest. 1992; 89: 1496-1500.

10. Satoh, T., Cohen, H.T., Katz, A.I. Intracellular signaling in the regulation of renal Na-K-ATPase: II. Role of eicosanoids. (manuscript submitted).

11. Torikai, S., Kurokawa, K. Effect of PGE_2 on vasopressin-dependent cell cAMP in isolated single nephron segments. Am J Physiol. 1983; 245: F58-F66.

12. Tria, E., Luly, P., Tomasi, V., Trevisani, A., Barnabei, O. Modulation by cyclic AMP in vitro of liver plasma membrane (Na^+-K^+)-ATPase and protein kinases. Biochim Biophys Acta. 1974; 343: 297-306.

13. Lingham, R.B., Sen, A.K. Regulation of rat brain (Na^+ + K^+)-ATPase activity by cyclic AMP. Biochim Biophys Acta. 1982; 688: 475-485.

14. Doucet, A. Multiple hormonal control of the Na/K-ATPase activity in the thick ascending limb. Proc Int Congress Nephrol. 1988; 10: 247-254.

15. Schwartzman, M., Ferreri, N.R., Carroll M.A., Songu-Mize, E., McGiff J.C. Renal cytochrome P450-related arachidonate metabolite inhibits (Na^++K^+)ATPase. Nature. (Lond.) 1985; 314: 620-622.

16. Hébert, R.L., Jacobson, H.R., Breyer, M.D. Prostaglandin E_2 inhibits sodium transport in rabbit cortical collecting duct by increasing intracellular calcium. J Clin Invest. 1991; 87: 1992-1998.

17. Hirata, F. The regulation of lipomodulin, a phospholipase inhibitory protein, in neutrophils by phosphorylation. J Biol Chem. 1981; 256: 7730-7733.

18. Flower, R.J., Blackwell, G.J. Anti-inflammatory steroids induce biosynthesis of a phospholipase A_2 inhibitor which prevents prostaglandin generation. Nature (Lond.) 1979; 278: 456-459.

19. Capdevila, J., Gil, L., Orellana, M., Marnett, L.J., Mason, J.I., Yadagiri, P., Falck, J.R. Inhibitors of cytochrome P-450-dependent arachidonic acid metabolism. Arch Biochem Biophys. 1988; 261: 257-263.

20. Bonvalet, J.-P., Pradelles, P., Farman, N. Segmental synthesis and actions of prostaglandins along the nephron. Am J Physiol. 1987; 253: F377-F387.

21. Cheval, L., Doucet, A. Measurement of Na-K-ATPase-mediated rubidium influx in single segments of rat nephron. Am J Physiol. 1990; 259: F111-F121.

22. Soltoff, S.P., Mandel, L.J. Amiloride directly inhibits the Na,K-ATPase activity of rabbit kidney proximal tubules. Science. 1983; 220: 957-959.

Anatomical Localization of Dopamine DA-1 Receptors in the Human Kidney: A Light Microscope Autoradiographic Study

F. Amenta*, A. Ricci[†], S. Escaf[‡] and J.A. Vega[§]

*Lab. Neuromorfologia Neuropatologia, Dip. to Sanità Publica e
Biol. Cellulare, Università "Tor Vergata", Roma, Italy
[†]Dip. to Scienze Cardiovascolari e Respiratorie, Università "La
Sapienza", Roma, Italy
[‡]Dep. to Urologia, Hospital "San Agustin", Aviles, Spain
[§]Dep. to Morfologia y Biologia Celular, Universidad de Oviedo,
Oviedo, Spain

Key Words: dopamine, kidney, DA-1 receptors, human

ABSTRACT

The anatomical localization of dopamine DA-1 receptor sites was analyzed in frozen sections of human kidney
using combined radioligand binding and autoradiographic
techniques. [3H]-SCH 23390 which was used as a ligand was
bound to sections of human kidney in a manner consistent
with the labeling of dopamine DA-1 receptors. The dissociation constant value was 3.8 nM and the maximum density
of binding sites was 143 fmol/mg protein. Light microscope autoradiography revealed the highest accumulation of
silver grains which correspond to [3H]-SCH 23390 binding
sites within the macula densa and proximal convoluted
tubules of the nephron. A lower density of silver grains
was noticeable in the following order: the ascending limb
of the nephric (Henle's) loop, the distal convoluted
tubules, the descending limb of the nephric loop as well
as the tunica media of the intrarenal artery branches. No
specific [3H]-SCH 23390 binding was noticeable within the
glomeruli or the epithelium of the collecting tubules.

Correspondence: Prof. Francesco Amenta, Dipartimento di
Sanità Pubblica e Biologia Cellulare, Via O. Raimondo
8, 00173 ROMA Italy.

INTRODUCTION

The infusion of dopamine in low doses to humans causes diuresis, natriuresis and vasodilation in the renal vascular tree. Moreover, it increases the glomerular filtration rate. Extensive evidence has demonstrated that the effects of dopamine on renal function are mediated through the interaction of the catecholamine with specific dopamine receptors rather than with adrenoceptors. The same effects as well as an increase in plasma renin activity were observed by infusing DA-1 receptor agonists to healthy subjects [4].

The functional characteristics and the biochemical properties of renal dopamine receptors have been recently investigated in several mammals including humans (for a review see [5]). From these studies the existence of two dopamine receptor subtypes in the mammalian kidney, namely DA-1 and DA-2 receptors has been demonstrated. Moreover, it has been shown that specific dopamine receptor agonists lead to changes in renal electrolyte excretion and haemodynamics [5]. The anatomical localization of dopamine DA-1 receptor sites has been investigated by light microscope autoradiography in the rat kidney [6-11], whereas only sparse information is available concerning the localization of these receptors in humans. The aim of our study was to analyze the density and pattern of dopamine DA-1 receptors in the human kidney using combined radioligand binding and autoradiographic techniques.

METHODS

Samples of renal cortex and medulla were obtained from male patients (n=10; age range 35-65 years) undergoing partial or total nephrectomy. The portions of the kidney used for the present study did not show signs of pathologic lesions. Specimens were washed in ice-cold 0.9% NaCl, reduced into small blocks including the renal cortex and medulla or the cortex or the medulla alone, and embedded in a cryoprotectant medium (OCT, Ames, IA, U.S.A.). OCT blocks were frozen in isopentane cooled in liquid nitrogen and stored at -80°C until use. Serial 8 μm thick sections were mounted on acid-washed microscope slides and air dried.

In the first part of this study the pharmacological characteristics and the DA-1 receptor profile of the binding of the radioligand to sections of human kidney were assessed according to the procedure detailed elsewhere [10-11]. Sections were incubated for 60 min. at 25°C using increasing concentration (0.1-8 nM) of [3H]-SCH 23390 (specific activity 85 Ci/mmol, Amersham Radiochemical Centre, Amersham, U.K.). Non-specific binding was defined by the presence in the incubation medium of [3H]-SCH 23390 plus 1μM (+)-butaclamol. At the end of incubation the slides were washed in ice-cold Tris HCl buffer (2 x 5 min), rinsed in distilled water and wiped onto scintillation vials which were counted in a Beckman scintillation spectrometer.

In the second part of the study the autoradiographic localization of [3H]-SCH 23390 binding sites was assessed by light microscope autoradiography. Sections of the human kidney were incubated for 60 min at 25°C with 5nM [3H]-SCH 23390 in the presence or in the absence of 1μM (+)-butaclamol to define non-specific binding. After incubation, sections were washed in ice-cold Tris-HCl buffer, rinsed in distilled water and air dried. Sections were processed for autoradiography by attaching to them Ilford K5 nuclear emulsion-coated coverslips [9-11].

The density of silver grains developed within the different portions of the human nephron and within the intrarenal branches of the renal artery was assessed by counting the number of silver grains developed in a 250 μm² area of [3H]-SCH 23390 autoradiographs. For further details see Amenta and Ricci [10].

RESULTS

[3H]-SCH 23390 was specifically bound to sections of the human kidney. The binding was time-, temperature- and

concentration-dependent (data not shown). Scatchard analysis of binding isotherms revealed that in the range of
concentrations of [3H]-SCH 23390 used, it was bound to a
single class of high affinity sites. The dissociation
constant (Kd) value was 3.8 ± 0.25 nM and the maximum
density of binding sites was 143 ± 7.8 fmol/mg protein.
The highest specific : non-specific binding ratio was
achieved with a 5 nM [3H]-SCH 23390 concentration. Using
this radioligand concentration, the specific binding
represented more than 60% of total binding.

The pharmacological profile of [3H]-SCH 23390 binding
to sections of human kidney was consistent with the
labeling of dopamine DA-1 receptors. In fact compounds
known to interact with DA-1 receptors or with a mixed DA-
1 and DA-2 receptor profile displaced [3H]-SCH 23390 from
sections of human kidney. In contrast compounds interacting with DA-2 receptors, with adrenoceptors or with
serotonin receptors were inactive or weak displacers of
[3H]-SCH 23390 (table 1).

Light microscope autoradiography revealed the accumulation of silver grains primarily within the renal cortex. The highest density of specific silver grains was
noticeable within the macula densa and proximal convoluted tubules followed in descending order by the ascending limb of the nephric (Henle's) loop, the distal
convoluted tubules and the descending limb of the nephric
loop (Fig.1). No specific [3H]-SCH 23390 binding was

TABLE   1.- Pharmacological specificity of [3H]-SCH   23390

binding to sections of human kidney

Compounds	Ki (nM)
Bromocriptine	>10,000
(+)-Butaclamol	0.98 ± 0.11
(-)-Butaclamol	931 ± 34
Domperidone	>10,000
Dopamine	321 ± 19
Fenoldopam	39 ± 1.12
Haloperidol	4.78 ± 0.27
Ketanserine	7,350 ± 324
Phentolamine	>10,000
(-)-Propranolol	>10,000
SCH 23390	0.28 ± 0.04
Serotonin	2,960 ± 185
(+)-Sulpiride	6.35 ± 0.41
(-)-Sulpiride	>10,000

[3H]-SCH 23390 binding to sections of human kidney was
assayed using a 5 nM radioligand concentration. Values
competitor dissociation represent the constant (Ki)   ±
S.E.M. of 3-6 triplicate experiments. The Ki value was
calculated using the formule $Ki = IC_{50}/(1) + s/Kd$, where
IC_{50} is the displacer concentration inhibiting 50% of
specific binding, S is the optimal concentration of [3H]-
SCH 23390 to obtain the highest specific/non-specific
binding ratio and Kd is the dissociation constant value.

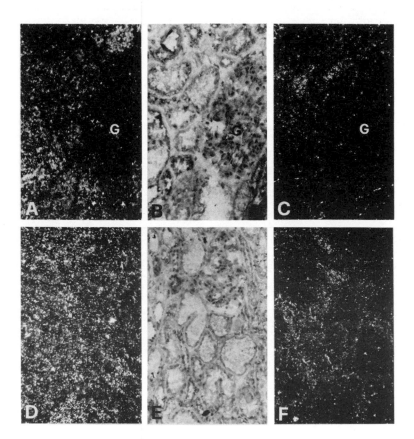

Fig. 1.- Autoradiographic localization of dopamine DA-1
receptor sites in the human renal cortex (A-C) and in the
epithelium of the nephric loop (D-E). Sections were
exposed to a 5 nM [3H]-SCH 23390 alone (pictures A and D)
or plus 1 μM (+)-butaclamol (pictures C and F) to cause
non-specific binding. Pictures A, C, D and F are dark-
field micrographs. Pictures B and E are bright-field
micrographs stained with toluidine blue to verify
microanatomical details. G = glomeruli. (x 125).

noticeable within glomeruli (Fig.1) or the epithelium of collecting tubules (data not shown).

Silver grains were also located in the tunica media of different sized renal artery intraparenchymal branches. No significant differences in the density of silver grains were noticeable between the tunica media of inter- lobular, arcuate or cortical radial arteries (data not shown).

DISCUSSION

By using combined radioligand binding and autoradio- graphic techniques with [3H]-SCH 23390 as a ligand, we have reported the existence of dopamine DA-1 receptor sites in several portions of the tubular component of the human nephron as well as within the intraparenchymal branches of the renal artery. The biochemical-pharmacolo- gical characterization of dopamine DA-1 receptors in the human kidney has been accomplished by measuring dopa- mine-dependent adenylate cyclase activity in membrane particulates of renal cortex [12] and the binding of the DA-1 receptor ligand [125I]-SCH 23390 to plasma membranes of the renal cortex [13]. However, as far as we know, this is one of the first reports identifying the detailed localization of dopamine DA-1 receptor sites in the human kidney [14]. The problem of the anatomical localization of dopamine receptors in the kidney may have functional relevance in view of the disagreement of investigators whether the diuretic and natriuretic effects of dopamine are secondary to renal vasodilation or dependent on a tubular action of the catecholamine and its agonists (for a review see [4]).

In the human kidney the localization of DA-1 receptor sites is similar to that already reported by other investigators and by some of us in the rat kidney [6-11]. The presence of DA-1 receptors within the epithelium of the nephric loop, has not been reported in the rat kidney [6-11]. Further studies are necessary to establish whether the existence of DA-1 receptors in the nephric loop represents a characteristic of the human species or if it is due to technical reasons. Moreover, independent of the existence of DA-1 receptor sites in the nephric loop of the rat, the demonstration of these receptors in the portion of the nephron where the transcellular transport of Na is involved in urine concentration [15] suggests a role of DA-1 receptors in the control of urine concentration.

A comparative analysis of the density of DA-1 receptors in the tubular portion of the nephron and in intrarenal vasculature shows similar to the rat kidney [10], a higher density of DA-1 recognition sites in the tubular rather than in the vascular component of the human kidney. These findings support the observation that dopamine and DA-1 receptor agonist infusion causes primarily natriuresis in man [4]. Moreover, they suggest that DA-1 receptors probably play a more important role in regula-

ting diuresis than haemodynamics

ACKNOWLEDGMENTS
    The present study was supported by grants of the Italian National Research Council (C.N.R.) and of "Tor Vergata" University and by a grant of F.I.S.S. (Spain) No.92/1014

REFERENCES

1. Golderg LI. The relationship of receptor actions of dopamine agonists to their clinical effects. In: Dopamine Receptor Antagonists. PG Crooke (ed.), Plenum Press, New York-London, pp. 291-301, 1985.

2. ter Wee PM, Smith AJ, Rosman JB, Sluiter WJ and Donker AJM. Effect of intravenous infusion of low-dose dopamine on renal function in normal individuals and in patients with renal disease. Am J Nephrol, 6: 42-46, 1986a.

3. ter Wee PM, van Ballegooie E, Rosman JB, Meijer S and Donker AJM. The effect of low-dose dopamine on renal haemodynamics in patients with Type I (insulin-dependent) diabets does not differ from normal individuals. Diabetologia, 29: 78-81, 1986b.

4. Girbes ARJ, Smith AJ, Meijer S and Rcitsma WD. Renal and endocrine effects of fenoldopam and metoclopramide in normal man. Nephron, 56: 179-185, 1990.

5. Lokhandwala MF and Amenta F. Anatomical distribution and function of dopamine receptors in the kidney. FASEB J, 5: 3023-3030, 1991.

6. Felder RA and Jose PA. Dopamine-1 receptors in rat kidneys identified with [125I]-SCH 23390. Am J Physiol, 255: F970-F976, 1988.

7. Hegde SS, Ricci A, Amenta F and Lokhandwala MF. Evidence from functional and autoradiographic studies for the presence of tubular dopamine-1 receptors and their involvement in the renal effects of fenoldopam. J Pharmacol Exp Ther, 251: 1237-1245, 1989.

8. Huo T and Healy PH. Autoradiographic localization of dopamine DA-1 receptors in the rat kidney with [3H]-SCH 23390. Am J Physiol, 257: F414-F423, 1989.

9. Amenta F. Biochemistry and autoradiography of

peripheral dopamine receptors. In: Peripheral Dopamine Pathophysiology. F Amenta (ed.), CRC Press, Boca Raton, pp. 39-51, 1990.

10. Amenta F and Ricci A. Autoradiographic localization of dopamine DA-1 receptors in the rat renal vasculature using [3H]-SCH 23390 as a ligand. J Autonom Pharmacol, 10: 371-381, 1990.

11. Amenta F and Ricci A. Demonstration of dopamine DA-1 receptor sites in rat juxtaglomerular cells by light microscope autoradiography. Naunyn-Schmiedeberg's Arch Pharmacol, 342: 719-721, 1990.

12. Baldi E, Pupilli C, Amenta F and Mannelli M. Presence of dopamine-dependent adenylate cyclase in human renal cortex. Eur J Pharmacol, 149: 351-356, 1988.

13. Hughes A and Sever P. Specific binding of [125I]-SCH 23982, a selective dopamine (D1) receptor ligand to plasma membranes derived from human kidney cortex. Biochem Pharmacol, 38: 781-785, 1989.

14. Amenta F. Density and distriution of dopamine receptors in the cardiovascular system and in the kidney. J Auton Pharmacol, 10, Suppl. 1: s10-s18, 1990.

15. Guyton AC. Textbook of Medical Physiology. Saunders, Phyladelphya, 1971.

Dopamine Receptor Modulation of Neurotransmission in Rat and Human Kidney

L.C. Rump and P. Schollmeyer

Innere Medizin IV, Universitätsklinik Freiburg, Hugstetter Str. 55,
W-7800 Freiburg, Germany

ABSTRACT

Modulation of neurotransmission by prejunctional dopamine receptors was investigated in human and rat kidney. In human renal cortex D_2-receptor activation by quinpirole but not D_1-receptor activation by fenoldopam inhibits noradrenaline release. The recently developed D_2-receptor agonist carmoxirole also inhibits noradrenaline release via activation of prejunctional D_2-receptors in human renal cortex. However, carmoxirole fails to inhibit noradrenaline release in rat isolated kidney due to simultaneous blockade of inhibitory α-autoreceptors. The inhibitory D_2-receptor mediated effect of carmoxirole in rat kidney can only be seen when prejunctional α-autoreceptors are functionally eliminated by phentolamine. This suggests that the α-adrenoceptor blocking activity of carmoxirole is more prominent in rat isolated kidney than in human renal cortex. D_2-receptor activation by quinpirole inhibits noradrenaline release and pressor responses to renal nerve stimulation in rat isolated kidney. The inhibitory effect of quinpirole on pressor responses is a consequence of its prejunctional effect since it does not inhibit pressor responses to exogenous noradrenaline. Phentolamine resistant pressor responses in rat kidney seem to be due to ATP which is coreleased with noradrenaline. D_2-receptor agonists reduce these purinergic pressor responses by inhibiting neuronal ATP release via activation of prejunctional D_2-receptors.

INTRODUCTION

Activation of dopamine receptors on postganglionic sympathetic nerve endings inhibits noradrenaline release (1) whereas activation of dopamine receptors on vascular smooth muscle cells mediates vasodilatation in a wide variety of tissues (2). These dopamine receptors have been classified as D_1-and D_2-receptors based on a potency range of various dopaminergic agonists and antagonists (3). In general, D_1-receptors are located postjunctionally and D_2-receptors prejunctionally. Prejunctional inhibitory D_2-receptors seem to be present on rabbit (4), dog (5) and rat (6, 7, 8) renal sympathetic nerves. The aim of the present study was to test as to whether D_1- and D_2-receptor agonists modulate noradrenaline release from human renal sympathetic nerves. Since an enhanced sympathetic nerve activity of the kidney seems to play an important role in hypertension (9), the effect of the recently developed, potentially antihypertensive D_2-receptor agonist carmoxirole (10) on noradrenaline release from superfused human renal cortex was also investigated. The rat isolated kidney preparation was used for comparison.

METHODS

Kidneys of Wistar rat were isolated and perfused with Krebs-Henseleit solution at a constant rate of 6 ml/min as previously described (8). The use of human renal cortex was approved by the local ethics committee. Human renal cortex was taken from patients undergoing surgery because of hypernephroma. Cortical kidney slices were prepared and superfused in superfusion chambers at a rate of 1.8 ml/min with Krebs-Henseleit solution as previously described (11). After incubation with $(-)-[2,5,6-^3H]$-noradrenaline human renal cortex slices and rat isolated kidneys were superfused (perfused) with drug free Krebs-Henseleit solution to remove loosely bound radioactivity. After the washing, consecutive samples of the superfusate (perfusate) were collected in 3 min fractions. There were two stimulation periods S_1 and S_2 (human kidney: 27 min apart, 5 Hz, 1 ms duration, 60s; rat kidney: 30 min apart, 50 V, 1 ms duration, 30 s). At the end of the experiments total tissue radioactivity of each kidney slice was determined. The stimulation induced (S-I) outflow of radioactivity was measured in the superfusate (perfusate) and in the case of human kidney slices subsequently expressed as a fraction of the total tissue radioactivity at the time of stimulation (fractional S-I outflow, FR). S-I outflow of radioactivity in S_2 and S-I pressor responses in S_2 are expressed as a percentage of the respective values in S_1. The effect of drugs was tested by adding them to the superfusion (perfusion) solution 12 min before S_2. When a drug was present throughout (th) the whole experiment, it was added to the superfusion solution 30 min before S_1. The Krebs-Henseleit solution had the following composition (mM): NaCl, 118; KCl, 4.7; $CaCl_2$, 2.5; $MgSO_4$, 0.45, $NaHCO_3$, 25; KH_2PO_4, 1.03; D-(+)-glucose, 11.1; disodium edetate, 0.067, ascorbic acid, 0.07. The following drugs were purchased: Levo-[ring-2,5,6-^{3}H]noradrenaline (NEN, Dreieich, FRG). Phentolamine (Ciba-Geigy, Wehr, FRG). α,ß-methylene ATP (Sigma, St. Louis, USA). S(-)-sulpiride and SCH 23390 (R(+)-7-chloro-8-hydroxy-3-methyl-1-phenyl-2,3,4,5,tetrahydro-1H-3-benzazepine (Biotrend, Cologne, FRG). Carmoxirole (EMD 45609; Merck, Darmstadt, FRG) and fenoldopam (Dr. Szabo, Pharmakologisches Institut, Universität Freiburg) were generous gifts.

RESULTS

Effects of D_1-and D_2-Receptor Agonists on S-I Outflow of Radioactivity from Human Renal Cortex Preincubated with ^{3}H-noradrenaline at 5 Hz.

The D_2-receptor agonists quinpirole (1 μM) and carmoxirole (0.03 μM) inhibited S-I outflow of radioactivity and both effects were unaltered by the non-selective α-adrenoceptor antagonist phentolamine (1 μM) (Fig 1). The D_1-receptor agonist fenoldopam (1 μM) enhanced S-I outflow of radioactivity but was without an effect in the presence of phentolamine (Fig 1). The D_2-receptor antagonist S(-)-sulpiride (10 μM) but not the D_1-receptor antagonist SCH 23390 (1 μM) blocked the inhibitory effects of quinpirole and carmoxirole (Fig 1).

Effect of D_2-receptor Agonists and α,ß-Methylene ATP on Neurotransmission in Rat Isolated Kidney at 1 Hz.

Quinpirole (0.3 μM) inhibited S-I outflow of radioactivity (Fig 2) and S-I pressor responses (Fig 2). Both effects were reversed by S(-)-sulpiride (10 μM) (Fig 2). The inhibitory effect of quinpirole was unaltered by phentolamine (1 μM) (Fig 2). Quinpirole (0.3 μM) did not inhibit pressor responses to exogenous noradrenaline (data not shown). The P_{2x}-receptor desensitizing agent α,ß-methylene ATP (mATP) did not modulate S-I outflow of radioactivity in the presence of phentolamine (Fig 2). Phentolamine resistant pressor responses were inhibited by quinpirole and by mATP (Fig 2). Carmoxirole (0.03 μM) failed to inhibit S-I outflow of radioactivity (91.1 $\pm$ 3.8 %, n=4) as compared to control (95.1 $\pm$ 3.6, n=7). However, in the presence of

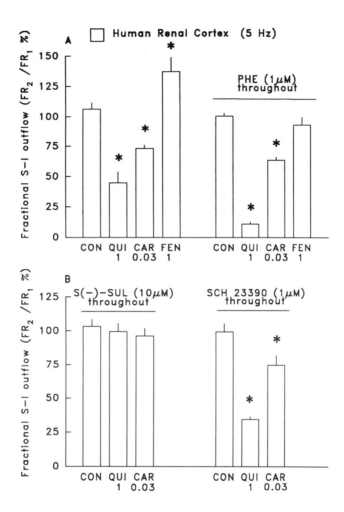

Fig 1 Effect of quinpirole (QUI), carmoxirole (CAR) and fenoldopam (FEN) on fractional S-I outflow of radioactivity from human kidney slices incubated with ^{3}H-noradrenaline. 1(A). In the absence of other drugs: Control (CON, n=20), QUI (1 μM, n=5), CAR (0.03 μM, n=6), FEN (1 μM, n=8). 2(A). Phentolamine (PHE) present throughout (th): CON (n=9), CAR (0.03 μM, n=5), FEN (1 μM, n=8). 3 (B). S(-)sulpiride (S(-)-SUL) present (th): CON (n=5), QUI (1 μM, n=5), CAR (0.03 μM, n=5). 4(B). SCH 23390 present (th): CON (n=6), QUI (1 μM, n=5, CAR (0.03 μM, n=6). All data are mean ± SEM. * significant difference from control (Student's unpaired t-test, p < 0.05).

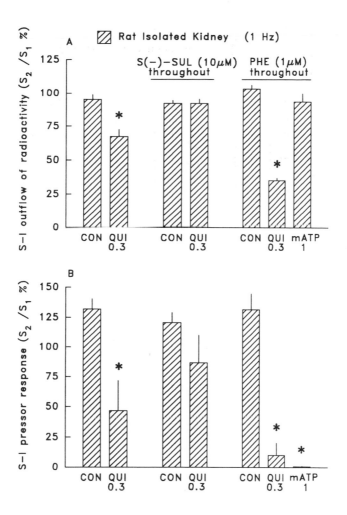

Fig 2 Effect of quinpirole (QUI) and α,ß-methylene ATP (mATP) on S-I outflow of radioactivity (A) and S-I pressor responses (B) in rat kidney incubated with ^{3}H-noradrenaline. 1. In the absence of other drugs: 1. Control (CON, n=7), QUI (0.3 μM, n=4). 2. S(-)-sulpiride (S(-)-SUL) present throughout (th): CON (n=4), QUI (0.3 μM, n=5). 3. Phentolamine (PHE) present (th): CON (n=6), QUI (0.3 μM, n=4), mATP (1 μM, n=4). All data are mean ± SEM. * significant difference from control (Student's unpaired t-test, p < 0.05).

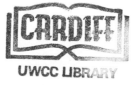

phentolamine (1 μM) carmoxirole (0.03 μM) inhibited S-I outflow of radioactivity (62.7 $\pm$ 7.5 %, n=5) and S-I pressor responses (data not shown) as compared to control (103.6 $\pm$ 2.7, n=6).

DISCUSSION

Human cortical kidney slices and rat isolated kidneys were incubated with ^{3}H-noradrenaline. The S-I outflow of radioactivity from sympathetically innervated tissues (12) including human renal cortex (13) can be taken as an index of endogenous noradrenaline release. In human renal cortex the D_2-receptor agonists quinpirole (1 μM) and carmoxirole (0.03 μM) inhibited S-I outflow of radioactivity. The inhibitory effect of both drugs is most likely due to activation of prejunctional D_2-receptors, since it was blocked by the selective D_2-receptor antagonist S(-)-sulpiride but not by the selective D_1-receptor antagonist SCH 23390. Sympathetic nerve endings of human renal cortex possess also prejunctional inhibitory α-autoreceptors, which, when activated by the α_2-adrenoceptor agonist UK 14304, mediate inhibition of noradrenaline release (13). However, an effect of quinpirole (1 μM) and carmoxirole (0.03 μM) on prejunctional α-adrenoceptors seems unlikely, since the inhibitory effects of quinpirole and carmoxirole (0.03 μM) were not prevented by the non-selective α-adrenoceptor antagonist phentolamine, whereas the inhibitory effect of UK 14304 was totally abolished by phentolamine (13). The D_1-receptor agonist fenoldopam (1 μM) facilitated S-I outflow of radioactivity from human renal cortex. Drugs can increase S-I outflow of radioactivity from tissues incubated with ^{3}H-noradrenaline either by activating prejunctional facilitatory receptors (e.g. ß-adrenoceptors or angiotensin II receptors) or more indirectly by blocking inhibitory autoreceptors. Since the facilitatory effect of fenoldopam was not seen in the presence of phentolamine, it seems rather to be due to blockade of prejunctional α-autoreceptors than to activation of prejunctional D_1-receptors. In rat isolated kidney quinpirole (0.3 μM) inhibited S-I outflow of radioactivity. This effect was blocked by S(-)- sulpiride but neither by SCH 23390 nor by phentolamine. Similar data have been obtained previously (7). Quinpirole had no effect on pressor responses to exogenous noradrenaline but inhibited pressor responses to renal nerve stimulation, which have been shown to be largely sensitive to the α_1-adrenoceptor antagonist prazosin (8). This suggests that activation of prejunctional D_2-receptors in rat kidney inhibits noradrenaline release and thereby reduces pressor responses to renal nerve stimulation. Surprisingly, carmoxirole (0.03 μM) failed to inhibit S-I outflow of radioactivity in rat kidney. However, this lack of inhibition seems to be due to simultaneous blockade of α-autoreceptors, since in the presence of phentolamine carmoxirole (0.03 μM) inhibited S-I outflow of radioactivity. Higher concentrations of carmoxirole (0.3 μM) show an even more pronounced α-adrenoceptor blocking effect in rat (8) and also human kidney (13). Co-release of noradrenaline and ATP from sympathetic nerves has been demonstrated in various tissues (14) including the kidney (15, 16). Moreover, blockade of prejunctional α-autoreceptors increases not only the release of noradrenaline but also that of ATP (14). Pressor responses to renal nerve stimulation in rat kidney in the presence of pre- and postjunctional α-adrenoceptor blockade by phentolamine were abolished by the P_{2X}-desensitizing agent α,β-methylene ATP, which by itself did not alter S-I outflow of radioactivity. Thus, pressor responses at 1 Hz in rat kidney in the presence of phentolamine seem to be entirely due to an enhanced release of ATP. Since phentolamine resistant pressor responses were also inhibited by quinpirole and carmoxirole, it is suggested, that activation of prejunctional D_2-receptors inhibits the co-release of ATP from sympathetic nerves in rat kidney.

ACKNOWLEDGEMENTS

The work in the author's laboratory is supported by a grant of the Deutsche Forschungsgemeinschaft (Ru 401/1-2). We thank the Ms U. Schaible for expert technical assistance and the Dept. of Urology (Prof.Sommerkamp) for the supply of human renal tissue.

REFERENCES

1. Willems, J.L., Buylaert, W.A., Bogaert, M.G. Neuronal dopamine receptors on autonomic ganglia and sympathetic nerves in the gastrointestinal system. Pharmacol Rev. 1985; 37: 165-216.

2. Brodde, O.E. Vascular dopamine receptors: demonstration and characterization by in vitro studies. Life Sci. 1982; 31: 289-306.

3. Hilditch, A., Drew, G.M. Peripheral dopamine receptor subtypes - a closer look. Trends Pharmacol Sci. 1985; 6: 396-400.

4. Chevillard, C., Mathieu, M.N., Recommis, D. Prejunctional actions of piribedil on the isolated kidney of the rabbit: comparison with apomorphine. Br J Pharmacol. 1980; 71: 513-518.

5. Bass, A.S., Robie, N.W. Stereoselectivity of S- and R-sulpiride for pre- and postsynaptic dopamine receptors in the canine kidney. J Pharmacol Exp Ther. 1984; 229: 67-71.

6. Lokhandwala, M.F., Steenberg, M.L. Selective activation by LY 141865 and apomorphine of presynaptic dopamine receptors in rat kidney and influence of stimulation parameters in the action of dopamine. J Pharmacol Exp Ther. 1984; 228: 161-167.

7. Lokhandwala, M.F., Steenberg, M.L. Evaluation of the effects of SKF 82526 and LY 171555 on presynaptic (DA_2) and postsynaptic (DA_1) dopamine receptors in rat kidney. J Auton Pharmac, 1984; 4: 273-277.

8. Rump, L.C., Wilde, K., Bohmann, C., Schollmeyer P. Effects of the novel DA_2-receptor agonist carmoxirole (EMD 45609) on noradrenergic and purinergic neurotransmission in rat isolated kidney. Naunyn Schmiedeberg's Arch Pharmacol. 1992; 345: 300-308.

9. Katholi, R.E. Renal nerves and the pathogenesis of hypertension in experimental animals and humans. Am J Physiol. 1983; 245: F1-F14.

10. Hauesler, G. Potential future developments in the field of antihypertensive drugs. Eur Heart J [Suppl. M]. 1987; 8: 135-142.

11. Rump L.C., Schuster, M.J., Schollmeyer, P. Activation of β_2-adrenoceptors by isoprenaline and adrenaline enhances noradrenaline release in cortical kidney slices of young spontaneously hypertensive rats. Naunyn Schmiedeberg's Arch Pharmacol. 1992; 345: 25-32.

12. Starke, K. Regulation of noradrenaline release by presynaptic receptor systems. Rev Physiol Biochem Pharmacol. 1977; 77: 1-124.

13. Rump, L.C., Schwertfeger, E., Schuster, M.J., Schaible, U., Frankenschmidt, A., Schollmeyer, P. Dopamine DA_2-receptor activation inhibits noradrenaline release in human kidney slices . Kidney Int (submitted).

14. Von Kügelgen, I., Starke, K. Noradrenaline-ATP-co-transmission in the sympathetic nervous system. Trends Pharmacol Sci. 1991; 12: 319-324.

15. Schwartz, D.D., Malik, K. U. Renal nerve stimulation-induced vasoconstriction at low frequencies is primarily due to release of a purinergic co-transmitter in the rat. J Pharmacol Exp Ther. 1989; 250: 764-771.

16. Rump, L.C., Wilde, K., Schollmeyer, P. Prostaglandin E_2 inhibits noradrenaline release and purinergic pressor responses to renal nerve stimulation at 1 Hz in isolated kidneys of young spontaneously hypertensive rats. J Hypertens. 1990; 8: 897-908.

Effects of Dopamine Agonists on Sympathetic Nervous System

J.L. Montastruc, C. Damase-Michel, G. Durrieu,
M.A. Tran and P. Montastruc

Laboratoire de Pharmacologie Médicale et Clinique, INSERM U317,
Faculté de Médecine, 37 allées Jules-Guesde, 31073 Toulouse Cédex,
France

ABSTRACT

Dopamine (DA) receptor agonists have a potential therapeutic interest in several cardiovascular diseases (hypertension, heart failure...). However, their effect on the activity of the sympathetic nervous system remains discussed. The present study investigates the effects of several selective DA1 and DA2 agonists on the release of catecholamines under three different conditions :

1° *"In vitro" studies* : quinpirole, a DA2 agonist, but not fenoldopam, a DA1 agonist, decreased noradrenaline and dopamine (but not adrenaline) release from dog renal cortical slices suggesting the potential involvement of DA2 receptors in the control of noradrenergic neurotransmission in the kidney.

2° *"In vivo" studies* : the effects of several DA agonists were studied in three groups of conscious dogs : normal dogs, animals made hypertensive by sinoaortic denervation (this model allows to investigate changes in sympathetic tone independently of baroreflex involvement) and dogs with diabetes insipidus. Quinpirole exerts both a peripheral depressor action (which explains the decrease in blood pressure) and a central pressor component involving an increase in sympathetic tone. Moreover, quinpirole (or apomorphine) did not directly modify adrenal catecholamine release.

3° *Clinical studies* : in patients with Parkinson's disease, a chronic treatment with the DA2 agonist bromocriptine alone (but not levodopa + dopa-decarboxylase inhibitor) decreased plasma catecholamine levels. Bromocriptine and levodopa blunted the sympathetic response to standing up.

In conclusion, the effects of DA agonists on sympathetic nervous system appear to be rather complex. These drugs first increase sympathetic tone through central and baroreflex mechanisms. On the other hand, the activation of peripheral DA2 receptors evoked a fall in blood pressure due to the decrease in noradrenaline release from vascular and renal sympathetic nerve endings. Moreover, DA agonists do not directly modify catecholamine release from the adrenal gland suggesting that peripheral DA receptors are not involved in the control of adrenal catecholamine release under "in vivo" conditions.

INTRODUCTION

The involvement of dopamine (DA) receptors in the regulation of blood pressure is well established. However, conflicting results were reported in the literature (1). In fact, DA and other DA receptor agonists may affect blood pressure either by direct renal vasodilatation through stimulation of specific postjunctional DA receptors or by inhibition of the release of noradrenaline from peripheral noradrenergic nerve terminals, through the stimulation of prejunctional DA receptors or by direct stimulation of central dopamine pre- or postsynaptic receptors. Thus, according to experimental procedures, the administration of a DA agonist either leads to a decrease (2, 3) or an increase (4, 5) in blood pressure and heart rate. The respective involvement of central and peripheral mechanisms in both cardiovascular responses and catecholamine release after administration of DA compounds remains to be investigated. Thus, the effects of several selective DA agonists on sympathetic tone were studied under three different conditions : *"in vitro"* (dog renal cortical slices), *"in vivo"* (hemodynamic studies in conscious dogs) and clinical studies (patients with Parkinson's disease).

"IN VITRO" STUDIES

The effects of DA agonists on the renal catecholamine release were investigated on dog kidney slices. Quinpirole (10^{-6} M to 10^{-3}M), a DA2 selective agonist, or fenoldopam (10^{-6}M), a DA1 agonist, were directly added to the incubation medium containing dog renal cortical slices. Quinpirole (but not fenoldopam) decreased noradrenaline and dopamine release whereas adrenaline release remained unchanged.

These preliminary results suggest the potential involvement of DA2 receptors in the control of renal sympathetic tone. In fact, such an inhibitory effect of DA2 agonists on noradrenaline release had been previously described on ganglionic receptors of the sympathetic nervous system (6, 7, 8). DA2 receptors were also described on renal homogenates (9, 10, 11, 12, 13, 14, 15, 16, 17) on basolateral and brush border membranes of renal tubular cells (18), on rat glomerulus (19) in inner medullary collecting duct (20). Radioreceptor binding and autoradiographic studies have allowed to identify DA2 receptor sites in the rat kidney (21). Until recently no data have provided a direct evidence for a functional role of renal DA2 receptors (22, 23). However, a recent study in the rat shows that quinpirole inhibits stimulation-induced outflow of noradrenaline and pressor responses to renal nerve stimulation. These effects were blocked by sulpiride (24). Taken together, these results and the present data suggest the involvement of DA2 receptors in the control of noradrenergic neurotransmission in the kidney.

"IN VIVO" STUDIES

In order to further characterize the overall *"in vivo"* effects of DA2 stimulation, we studied the effects of quinpirole in three groups of conscious dogs: (a) normotensive dogs,(b) animals made hypertensive by sinoaortic denervation (this model allowing to investigate changes in sympathetic tone independently of baroreflex involvements (25)) and (c) dogs with diabetes insipidus (i.e. animals deprived of vasopressin) (26).

In normotensive dogs, acute intravenous injection of quinpirole induced an increase in sympathetic tone (as shown by the rise in plasma catecholamine levels) associated with different changes in arterial blood pressure according to the experimental protocol. These observations explain the discrepancies reported in the literature after DA2 stimulation with quinpirole (1). In fact, several studies found a fall in both blood pressure and heart rate (2, 3), whereas Nagahama et al., (4) described a simultaneous rise in these two parameters. In normotensive dogs, different pattern of pressor and cardiac responses can be observed: in normal awake dogs, an hypotensive effect is associated with a positive chronotropic response. When compared with normal dogs, the hypotensive response was more pronounced *in sinoaortic denervated dogs*. In these sinoaortic denervated animals, the rise in heart rate was always present although less marked. These results suggest the involvement of both baroreflex pathways and central mechanisms in the tachycardic response elicited by quinpirole. The more marked depressor response observed after quinpirole in sinoaortic denervated dogs can be explained by both the high resting level of blood pressure (law of the initial level) and the absence of compensatory responses from baroreflex origin. Thus, the involvement of a central excitatory component in the cardiovascular effects of quinpirole administered by intravenous route can be suggested. This central mechanism can explain (at least partly) the tachycardia elicited by the DA2 agonist.

This last hypothesis was further tested by performing two kinds of experiments : first, i.c.m. (intra cisterna magna) injections of quinpirole ; secondly, i.c.m. injection of quinpirole after preatment with peripheral administration of domperidone, a selective DA2 antagonist deprived of any central effect (27). Under these two conditions, quinpirole induced an increase in both blood pressure and heart rate (25), confirming the central origin of the excitatory effects of quinpirole.

Beside this central effect, quinpirole also possesses peripheral depressor properties, as previously reported by several authors. In fact, peripheral stimulation of prejunctional or ganglionic dopamine receptors is known to induce a fall in blood pressure (6,7). However, in normal or sinoaortic denervated dogs, this hypotensive response is accompanied by an increase in plasma levels of catecholamines. How can we explain this apparent inconsistency : decrease in blood pressure with increased levels in plasma catecholamines ? One can hypothetized that both central and peripheral mechanisms are involved : in fact, the experiments with domperidone reported above have shown that the blockade of peripheral dopamine receptors reverses the depressor effect of quinpirole into a pressor effect. Thus, without central participation, the hypotensive effects would be more marked. In normal conscious dogs, the hypotensive component is predominant. By contrast, in normotensive rats, Nagahama et al. (4) observed a pressor response.

Intravenous administration of quinpirole induces a more marked decrease in blood pressure in conscious dogs with surgically-induced **diabetes insipidus** than in normal dogs. Moreover, the specific DA2 receptor agonist increased vasopressin plasma levels in normal dogs (figure 1) (28). Taken together, these results suggest the involvement of vasopressin in the changes in blood pressure observed after quinpirole. They clearly demonstrate that acute administration of quinpirole in normal dogs

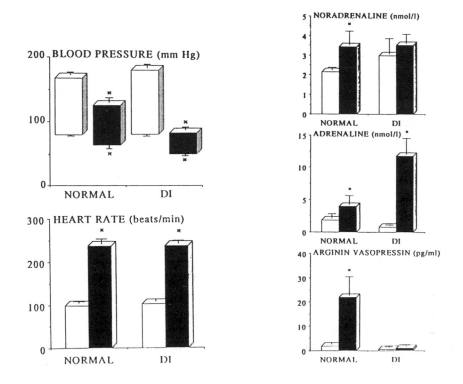

Figure 1 : Effect of intravenous administration of quinpirole (30 µg/kg)   on cardiovascular parameters (right pannel: blood pressure in mmHg, heart rate in beats/min), catecholamines and vasopressin plasma levels (left pannel) measured before (open columns) and 5 min after (solid columns) quinpirole injection in two groups of conscious dogs : normotensive controls (n = 6) and animals with diabetes insipidus (DI : n = 6). Statistical analysis was done with the Wilcoxon test for paired comparisons. Mean values are given. Vertical lines show S.E.M. * = p < 0.05 when compared with pretreatment values.

is associated with a rise in vasopressin release, which counteracts the hypotensive action of the DA2 agonist.

The increase in vasopressin plasma levels after quinpirole requires comment. First, the rise is not from baroreflex origin but probably results from central activation : in fact, an effect through baroreflex pathways can be ruled out since quinpirole still induces an increase in vasopressin plasma levels in sinoaortic denervated dogs. Thus, a central mechanism can be hypothetized since central administration of quinpirole at doses ineffective by peripheral route induces an increase in vasopressin levels in conscious dogs. Secondly, the results suggest the involvement of DA2 receptors in the increase in vasopressin levels. In fact, conflicting results about the involvement of these DA2 receptors in the control of vasopressin release have been reported in the literature. For instance, Nagahama et al. (29) described an increase in vasopressin plasma levels after quinpirole injection in rats. Morphological studies indicate that DA neurons terminate in the supraoptic nucleus, medium eminence and the neural lobe of the posterior pituitary (30). In contrast, Chiodera et al. (31) show that metoclopramide increases vasopressin release in humans. This last conflicting result can be explained by the lack of selectivity of metoclopramide, which is a mixed DA1/DA2 receptor antagonist. Under our experimental conditions, the increase in vasopressin in normal dogs is associated with a rise in plasma noradrenaline and adrenaline as a result of both baroreflex and central activation of sympathetic pathways. The rise in noradrenaline plasma levels was not found in dogs with diabetes insipidus. Thus, it is likely that vasopressin participates in the rise of noradrenaline plasma levels through an increase in sympathetic tone, as previously suggested by Share (32). This observation explains why quinpirole failed to increase noradrenaline levels in dogs with diabetes insipidus. We suggested that the dramatic decrease in blood pressure elicited by quinpirole in dogs with diabetes insipidus stimulates adrenaline release from the adrenal medulla.

This rise in sympathetic tone described in conscious dogs was also observed in anesthetized dogs (25). Thus, in conscious as well as in anesthetized dogs, the centrally mediated increase in sympathetic tone predominates over the peripheral depressor mechanism (i.e. the decrease in noradrenaline release from sympathetic nerve endings). In order to reveal this last peripheral component, we decided to work on *adrenal medulla* after section of the great splanchnic nerve because (a) adrenal medullary

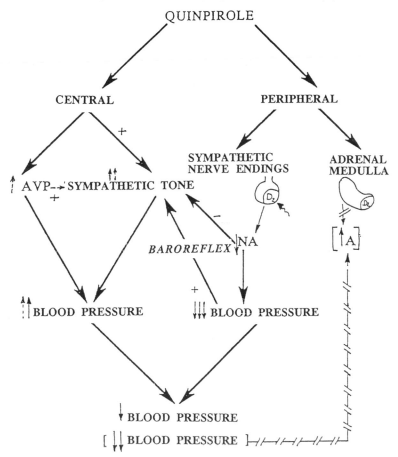

Figure 2 : Effects of quinpirole, a DA2 agonist, on sympathetic tone. Quinpirole induces both a central and peripheral effect leading to an increase in vasopressinergic and sympathetic tone. Adrenal medulla is not directly involved in the effect of quinpirole in normal animals. In dogs ith diabetic insipidus (hatched lines), the marked decrease in blood pressure (due to the absence of vasopressin : AVP) elicited an increased release in adrenaline (A) from adrenal medulla. NA : noradrenaline.

cells are embryologically analogous to sympathetic autonomic ganglia , (b) an effect of DA agonists on autonomic ganglia was postulated (8) and (c) *"in vitro"* experiments have identified DA2 receptors on adrenal medullary cells (33, 34). Moreover, apomorphine was previously found to inhibit the release of catecholamines from the perfused cat adrenal medulla, an effect which was reversed by haloperidol or sulpiride (35). Thus, the influence of apomorphine, a mixed DA1 and DA2 agonist, as well as quinpirole, a more selective DA2 agonist was investigated. Three different frequencies (1, 3 and 5 Hz) were used; for a 1 Hz frequency adrenal catecholamine secretion rates were almost identical with the basal values measured when adrenal nerve is intact. Moreover, according to Foucart et al. (36), the effects of drugs on splanchnic nerve stimulation could be dependent on the stimulation frequency. Under our experimental conditions, catecholamine release from the gland was frequency-dependent.

In the present *"in vivo"* study, it is important to note that apomorphine and quinpirole failed to reduce adrenal catecholamine release after nerve stimulation, whatever the frequencies of stimulation. In order to rigorously demonstrate the effects of drugs, we did not only use each animal as its own control but we compared the ratio S2/S1 between the values of the second stimulation (S2) and the corresponding values of the first period (S1) of electrical stimulation in the experimental (DA agonist-treated) group with the corresponding ratio values from the control (saline-treated) group. Under these conditions, basal resting values of adrenal catecholamines as well as adrenal plasma flow rates were unmodified when compared with control group (25).

Thus, the present data do not support the evidence for a physiological role of DA2 receptors in the *"in vivo"* control of adrenal medullary function.

In conclusion, quinpirole decreases blood pressure probably through a presynaptic inhibitory mechanism, as generally accepted. Moreover, we also describe an additional central pressor mechanism involving an increase in both sympathetic tone and vasopressin release (figure 2). These two effects can buffer the peripheral hypotensive action of quinpirole : the central property can be considered as a limiting factor in the potential therapeutic use of this group of drugs (DA2 agonists) in the treatment of arterial hypertension.

CLINICAL STUDIES

Blood pressure, heart rate, plasma noradrenaline and adrenaline levels in the lying and standing positions were compared in patients with Parkinson's disease (PD) and normal control subjects (37). Three groups of PD patients (Stage 2 and 3) were investigated : 6 patients deprived of antiparkinsonian drugs from 48 h, 7 levodopa + benserazide-treated patients and 7 bromocriptine-treated patients.   Blood pressure, heart rate and plasma catecholamines were similar at rest and in the standing position (an acurate procedure to investigate the reactivity of the autonomic nervous system) in controls and in PD patients deprived of antiparkinsonian drugs from 48 h. These results indicate that stages 2 to 3 of Parkinson's disease are not accompanied by major changes in autonomic cardiovascular function.

In these patients with PD, a chronic treatment with bromocriptine, a DA2 agonist (but not levodopa + dopamine decarboxylase inhibitor (DDI)) decreased plasma noradrenaline levels. Adrenaline plasma levels remained unchanged (37). These results suggest in agreement with other studies (38) that DA agonists decrease sympathetic tone mainly through a peripheral mechanism.

Moreover, both drugs (levodopa + DDI and bromocriptine) blunted the sympathetic response to standing up (37). This effect, which probably involves both central and peripheral mechanisms, explains the frequent occurence of orthostatic hypotension in PD patients treated with antiparkinsonian drugs (levodopa, DA ergot derivatives) (39).

CONCLUSION

The effects of DA agonists on sympathetic nervous system appear to be rather complex. *"In vivo"* studies show that these drugs first increase sympathetic and vasopressinergic tone through both central and baroreflex mechanisms. On the other hand, the activation of peripheral DA2 receptors evoked a fall in blood pressure due to the decrease in noradrenaline release from vascular and renal sympathetic nerve endings as demonstrated by *"in vitro"* and clinical studies in patients with Parkinson's disease. Finally, DA agonists do not directly modify catecholamine release from the adrenal gland suggesting that peripheral DA receptors are not involved in the control of adrenal catecholamine release under *"in vivo"* conditions.

REFERENCES

1. Montastruc, J.L., Damase-Michel, C., Montastruc, P. , Dopamine and hypertension. *In* Peripheral Dopamine Pathophysiology, ed. by F. Amenta, CRC Press, Boca Raton, FL, 163-169, 1989.
2. Cavero, I., Thirry, C., Pratz J. , Lawson, K. Cardiovascular characterization of DA1 and DA2 dopamine receptor agonists in anesthetized rats. Clin Exp Hypertension 1987 ; A9 : 931-952.
3. Hahn H.A., MacDonald, B.R., Martin, M.A. Primate cardiovascularresponses mediated by dopamine receptors : Effects of N,N-di-n-propyldopamine and LY171555. J. Pharmacol. Exp. Ther. 1984 ; 229 : 132-138.
4. Nagahama, S., Chen, Y.F., Lindheimer, M.D. , Oparil, S. : Mechanism of the pressor-action of LY 171555, a specific dopamine D2 receptor agonist in the conscious rat. J. Pharmacol Exp Ther. 1986 ; 236 : 735-742.
5. Kurtz, K., Main, B., Moore, R., Schmitt, T. : Differential effects of the selective dopamine (DA) agonist, quinpirole, on blood pressure in conscious normotensive and hypertensive rats. Fed Proc. 1986 ; 45 : 1071.
6. Langer, S.Z. : Presynaptic regulation of the release of catecholamines. Pharmacol Rev. 1981 ; 32 : 337-332.
7. Langer, S.Z. : Comparative analysis of presynaptic inhibition of noradrenaline release by alpha2 and dopamine receptors. Acta Pharmacol Toxicol. 1981 ; 49 : 20-21.
8. Willems, J.L., Buylaert, W.A., Lefebvre, R.A., Bogaert, M.G. Neuronal dopamine receptors on autonomic ganglia and sympathetic nerves and dopamine receptors in gastrointestinal system. Pharmacol Rev. 1985 ; 37 : 165-216.
9. Adam, W.R. Aldosterone and dopamine receptors in the kidney : sites for pharmacologic manipulation of renal function. Kidney Int. 1980 ; 18 : 623-635.
10. Felder, R.A., Blecher, M., Calcagno, P.L., Jose, P.A. Dopamine receptors in the proximal tubule of the rabbit. Am J Physiol. 1984 ; 247 : F499-F505.
11. Felder, R.A., Blecher, M., Eisner, G.M., Jose, P.A. Cortical tubular and glomerular dopamine receptors in the rat kidney. Am J Physiol. 1984 ; 246: F557-F568.
12. Felder, C.C., McKelvey, T.C., Blecher, M., Jose, P.A. Dopamine receptors (DA-R) in proximal tubular basolateral (BLM) and brush border membranes (BBM). Pediatr Res. 1987 ; 21 : 475.

13. Felder, R.A., Garland, D.S., José, P.A. Renal dopamine receptors in the spontaneously hypertensive rats (SHR). Pediatr Nephrol. 1987 ; 1 : C61.

14. Felder, R.A., José, P.A. Dopamine 1 receptors in rat kidneys identified with ^{125}I SCH 23982. Am J Physiol. 1988 ; 255 : F970-F976.

15. Nakajima, T. and Kurowa, I. Characterization with ^{3}H-haloperidol of the dopamine receptor in the rat kidney particulate preparation. Jap J Pharmacol. 1980 ; 30 : 891-898.

16. Rosenblatt, J.E., Shore,D., Wyatt, R .J., Pert, C.B. Increased renal neuroleptic binding in spontaneously hypertensive rats. Eur J Pharmacol. 1980 ; 67 : 317-320.

17. Shigetomi, S., Ueono, S., Tosaki, H., Kohno, H., Hashimoto, S., Fukuchi, S. Increased activity of sympatho-adrenomedullary system and decreased renal dopamine receptor content after short-term and long-term sodium loading in rats. Nippon-Naibunpi-Gakkai-Zasshi. 1986 ; 62 : 776-783.

18. Felder, C.C., McKelvey, A.M., Gitler, M.S., Eisner, G.M., Jose, P.A. Dopamine receptor subtypes in renal brushborder and basolateral membranes. Kidney Int. 1989 ; 36 : 183-193.

19. Felder, R.A. Autoradiographic localization of DA-1 dopamine receptors in microdissected rat proximal tubule. Kidney Int. 1987 ; 31 : 432.

20. Huo, T. and Healy, D.P. [^{3}H] Domperidone binding to the kidney inner medullary collecting duct dopamine-2K (DA 2K) receptor. J Pharmacol Exp Ther 1991 ; 258 : 424-428.

21. Amenta, F, Biochemistry and autoradiography of peripheral dopamine receptors. In Peripheral dopamine pathophysiology, ed. by F. Amenta, CRC Press, Boca Raton, FL, 163-169, 1989.

22. Frederickson, E.D., Bradley, D.T., Goldberg, L.I. Blockade of renal effects of dopamine in the dog by the DA1 antagonist SCH 23390. Am J Physiol. 1985; 249 : F236-F240.

23. Lokhandwala, M.F. and Hegde, S. Cardiovascular dopamine receptors : role of renal dopamine and dopamine receptors in sodium excretion. Pharmacol Toxicol. 1990 ; 66 : 237-243.

24. Rump, L.C., Wilde, K., Bohman, C., Schollmeyer, P. : Effects of the novel dopamine-receptor agonist carmoxirole (EMD 45609) on noradrenergic and purinergic neurotransmission in rat isolated kidney. Naunym Schmiedebergs' Arch Pharmacol. 1992 ; 345 : 300-308.

25. Damase-Michel, C., Montastruc, J.L., Gharib, C., Geelen, G., De Saint-Blanquat, G., Tran, M.A. : Effect of quinpirole, a specific dopamine DA2

receptor agonist on the sympathoadrenal system in dogs. J Pharmacol Exp Ther. 1990 ; 252 : 770-777.

26. Montastruc, J.L., Dang Tran, L., Castillo-Fernando, J.R., Morales-Olivas, F., Gaillard-Plaza, G., Montastruc P. : Effects of yohimbine and prazosin on water balance in dogs with diabetes insipidus. J Pharmacol (Paris). 1980; 11: 441.

27. Laduron, P.M. , Leysen, J.E. : Domperidone, a specific *in vitro* dopamine antagonist, devoid of *in vivo* central dopaminergic activity. Biochem Pharmacol. 1979 ; 28 : 2161-2165.

28. Damase-Michel, C., Montastruc, J.L., Tran, M.A., Gharib, C., Geelen,G.,Montastruc, P. : Involvement of vasopressin in the cardiovascular effects of quinpirole. Eur J Pharmacol. 1990 ; 184 : 179-183.

29. Nagahama, S., Ann, H.S., Chen, Y., Linheimer M.D., Oparil S. Role of vasopressin in the cardiovascular effects of LY 171555, a selective dopamine D2 receptor agonist : studies in conscious brattleboro and long-evans rats. J Pharmacol Exp Ther. 1987 ; 242 : 143.

30. Zaborsky L., Leranth, C., Maraka G.B., Palovits M. Quantitative studies on the supraoptic nucleus in the rat afferent fiber connections. Exp Brain Res. 1975 ; 22 : 525.

31. Chiodera, P., Volpi, R., Delsignore, R., Marchesi, R., C., Salati, G., Caminelli, L, Rossi, G., Coiro V. Different effects of metoclopramide and domperidone on arginine-vasopressin secretion in man. Br J Clin Pharmacol. 1986 ; 22 : 479.

32. Share, L. Role of vasopressin in cardiovascular regulation. Physiol. Rev. 1988; 68 : 1248.

33. Gonzalez, M.C., Artalejo, A.R., Montiel, C., Hervas P.P., Garcia, A.G. Characterization of a dopaminergic receptor that modulated adrenomedullary catecholamine release. J Neurochem. 1986 ; 47 : 382-388.

34. Lyon, R.A., Titeler, M., Bigornia, L. , D Schneider, A.S. D2 dopamine receptors on bovine chromaffin cell membranes : Identification and characterization by [3H]N-methylspiperone binding. J Neurochem. 1987 ; 48 : 631-635.

35. Artalejo, A.R., Garcia, A,G., Montiel C. , Sanchez-Garcia, P. A dopaminergic receptor modulates catecholamine release from the cat adrenal gland. J Physiol. (Lond.) 1985 ; 362 : 359-368.

36. Foucart, S., Lacaille-Belanger, P. Kimura, T., Nadeau R., De Champlain, J. Modulation of adrenal catecholamine release by DA2 dopamine receptors in the anesthetized dog. Clin Exp Pharmacol Physiol. 1988 ; 15 : 601-611.

37. Durrieu, G., Senard, J.M., Tran, M.A., Rascol, A., Montastruc, J.L. : Effects of levodopa and bromocriptine on blood pressure and plasma catecholamine in parkinsonians. Clin Neuropharmacol. 1991 ; 14 : 84-90.

38. Rascol, O., Montastruc, J.L. Cardiovascular effects of apomorphine in humans : evidence for peripheral mechanisms. Clin Neuropharmacol. 1986 ; 6 : 566-569.

39. Senard, J.M., Chamontin, B., Rascol A., Montastruc, J.L. :Ambulatory blood pressure in patients with Parkinson's disease without and with orthostatic hypotension. Clin Auton Res. 1992 ; 2 : 99-104.

Dopamine Receptor Stimulation During Exercise: Effects on Plasma Norepinephrine

A.R.J. Girbes[*,†], A.G. Lieverse[‡],
D.J. Van Veldhuisen[†], R.G. Grevink[§] and
A.J. Smit[†,‡]

[*]Division of Intensive Care of the Department of Surgery;
[†]Department of Cardiology; [‡]Internal Medicine; and [§]Pulmonology,
University Hospital Groningen, Oostersingel 59, 9713 EZ
Groningen, The Netherlands

ABSTRACT

We investigated the effects of 100 mg ibopamine, an orally active aselective dopamine agonist, on plasma catecholamines in 8 healthy males during graded exercise in a single blind, placebo controlled crossover study design. The exercise consisted of progressive cycling activity, up to 90% of the previously determined VO_2max. Graded exercise resulted in a rise of systolic- and mean blood pressure, heart rate, norepinephrine and epinephrine level, with a fall in diastolic blood pressure. The rise of norepinephrine was significantly blunted by ibopamine, compared with placebo. No differences for blood pressure, heart rate and epinephrine between the placebo- and ibopamine study day were found.

In previous studies ibopamine lowered resting plasma norepinephrine in patients with congestive heart failure, whereas plasma norepinephrine was not altered by ibopamine in healthy volunteers at rest. These effects of ibopamine might be ascribed to DA2-dopamine receptor mediated inhibition of norepinephrine release which only becomes manifest during active sympathetic stimulation like exercise or heart failure.

INTRODUCTION

The significance of plasma norepinephrine in clinical studies

Plasma norepinephrine is the net result of sympathetic activity spillover of the transmitter into the plasma and clearance from plasma. Therefore, the plasma norepinephrine level represents an indication of the sympathetic activity(1). Norepinephrine levels in patients with congestive heart failure and especially the influence of medical therapy on plasma norepinephrine levels have received increasing attention. Patients with (severe) congestive heart failure have an increased activity of the sympathetic nervous system and elevated norepinephrine levels at rest(1,2). In a recently published substudy of the Study Of Left Ventricular Dysfunction (SOLVD), neuroendocrine parameters of patients with left ventricular dysfunction (LVD) with and without symptoms of congestive heart failure (CHF) were determined and compared to normal controls (3). Two hundred and thirty-one patients with LVD were included: 150 without, called the prevention-group, and 81 with (called the treatment-group) CHF-symptoms. The median value for - among others - norepinephrine was significantly greater in the prevention-group than in the controls, whereas the value in the treatment-group was significantly greater than in the prevention-group. This indicates an early activation of the Sympathetic Nervous System (SNS). Furthermore, survival in patients with severe congestive heart failure is strongly related to norepinephrine levels(4). Swedberg et al. reported on the effects of ACE-inhibition on mortality when related to - among others - the level of plasma norepinephrine(5). This study was the report on the neuroendocrine data of the CONSENSUS trial, which studied the effect of ACE-inhibition on survival in patients with severe congestive heart failure. Patients were divided in two groups with levels **above** and **under** the median level of norepinephrine at the start of the treatment , respectively. Survival was better in the group with the lower values. Additionally, favorable changes of the survival-rate by medical treatment with an ACE-inhibitor were only achieved in patients with the higher initial norepinephrine levels. Although one may not conclude from this study that ACE-inhibition is only useful in patients with higher levels of norepinephrine, this study underlines the importance of potential modification of norepinephrine release in the chronic medical treatment of patients with congestive heart failure.

Norepinephrine release can be modulated presynaptically by different types of receptors: stimulation of (i) alpha-2 adrenoceptor or (ii) DA2-dopamine receptor results in inhibition of NE-release. Stimulation of beta-2 adrenoceptor and angiotensin-II receptor results in stimulation of NE-release. Beta-2 and angiotensin-II receptor antagonism will therefore lead to a decrease of norepinephrine release.

Dopamine agonists and plasma norepinephrine

Administration of oral dopamine agonists in patients with congestive heart failure has been associated with a fall in plasma norepinephrine levels. Both levodopa and bromocriptine have been shown to improve hemodynamics, accompanied by a fall in plasma norepinephrine, which was only sustained for bromocriptine(6,7). We and several other groups have shown that the new oral dopamine agonist ibopamine, a prodrug of methyl-dopamine (epinine), induces a fall in plasma norepinephrine in patients with heart failure(8-10).

In a recent study we have evaluated the renal hemodynamic effects of ibopamine in healthy man(11). As part of the study, plasma norepinephrine levels were measured at rest. No effects of ibopamine on plasma norepinephrine were found. Manelli et al.(12) indicated the importance of endogenous dopamine in limiting the rise of norepinephrine during exercise. We therefore hypothesized that a demonstrable effect of ibopamine on plasma norepinephrine might be present only during sympathetic stimulation, in the case of normal man: graded exercise.

METHODS: Dopamine receptor stimulation during exercise

Eight healthy men (31-38 years) were studied on three occasions. None was involved in formal exercise training during the preceding year. All studies were performed after a minimum of 3 h of fasting. After determination of the maximal oxygen consumption (VO_2max) on the second and third study day all subjects were submitted to graded exercise after ingestion of placebo or 100 mg ibopamine in random order. One week elapsed between each study day. After 15 minutes of supine rest, the first blood sample from a canula in the antebrachial vein, was drawn. Ibopamine or placebo was ingested, and after a further 30 minutes of supine rest, exercise was started at 30% of the predetermined VO_2max. The exercise load was increased every 3 minutes with steps of 10%, up to 90% of the VO_2max.

RESULTS

During exercise a rise in heart rate and systolic blood pressure, with a fall in diastolic bloodpressure was found. This was not influenced by ibopamine. The rise in epinephrine was not influenced by ibopamine. The effects of ibopamine on plasma norepinephrine during exercise are depicted in fig. 1.

DISCUSSION

In this study ibopamine blunted the exercise-induced rise of plasma norepinephrine in normal man. The most likely explanation is that ibopamine inhibits norepinephrine release by stimulation of presynaptic DA2-dopamine receptors. Another, although unlikely explanation for the blunting of plasma norepinephrine levels by ibopamine during sympathetic stimulation might be changes in forearm bloodflow. Since the concentration of venous plasma norepinephrine is a function of the inflowing not-extracted arterial norepinephrine, the net norepinephrine influx from local release sites, and the forearm bloodflow, any changes in blood-flow induced by ibopamine would affect the plasma level of norepinephrine. However, any possible changes in local hemodynamics induced by ibopamine would be negligible compared to the exercise induced changes in healthy volunteers, and one should expect more pronounced differences in plasma norepinephrine concentration at rest. Similarly, the contribution of a possible increase in cardiac output due to ibopamine is unlikely. Therefore, the effect on norepinephrine strongly suggests a DA2-receptor mediated effect of ibopamine. Apparently, this effect of ibopamine is detectable only during sufficient sympathetic stimulation. Similarly, endogenous dopamine plays a role in the control of norepinephrine release during sympathetic stimulation. In a study by Manelli et al.(12), the effects of DA2-receptor blockade by domperidone during sympathetic stimulation were

NOREPINEPHRINE

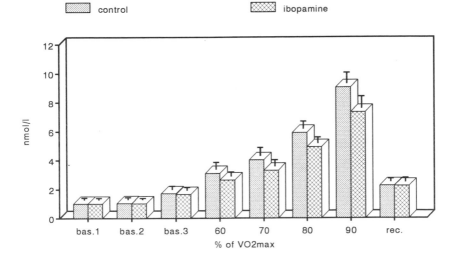

FIG.1 Plasma norepinephrine levels during exercise. A significant difference between the placebo and ibopamine is present at 80 and 90% of VO_2max. ($p<0.05$). bas.1: baseline, after 15 min supine rest; bas.2, baseline, 30 min after ibopamine ingestion; bas.3, baseline, 40 min after ibopamine ingestion, under resting sitting conditions; rec., recovery phase, after 3 min of 30% VO_2max and 5 min of complete sitting rest.

evaluated in seven healthy men in a double-blind randomized study. Graded exercise caused significant increases in - among others - plasma norepinephrine and epinephrine levels. Administration of 20 mg domperidone i.v. before graded exercise significantly enhanced the increase in plasma norepinephrine at the end of the exercise and resulted in an overall increase in plasma epinephrine levels compared to a control exercise study, while the increase in systolic and mean arterial blood pressure and in lactate levels was not affected by domperidone. The authors concluded that endogenous dopamine limits excessive adrenomedullary and neuronal catecholamine release. Preliminary results from a recently performed study - in our institution - in 10 healthy men show that 3 μg/kg/min dopamine i.v. also blunts the rise of norepinephrine, but only at 90% of the VO_2max, which was reversed by domperidone. At 70% of the VO_2max dopamine induced an increase of norepinephrine. Possibly the uptake1-inhibitive effect of dopamine plays a role in this respect.

In patients with heart failure, ibopamine blunted the increase of norepinephrine as well(13). The same effect, but mediated through another mechanism was observed in patients treated with the ACE-inhibitor captopril. Whereas the phosphodiesterase inhibitor milrinone produced similar short-term clinical improvement, but did not induce a reduction in plasma norepinephrine response to submaximal exercise(14).

We suppose that these neuroendocrine modifying effects may play a role in the improvement of survival in patients with heart failure. For ACE-inhibition beneficial effects on survival have been substantiated by clinical trials. We eagerly await similar studies with dopamine agonists.

ACKNOWLEDGEMENT

The authors want to thank Mrs. Annette Wiersma and Miss Brenda Aalders for their skillfull help in performing the studies.

REFERENCES

1. Cuche, J.L. Noradrénaline plasmatique. Signification et intérêt pratique de son dosage. Presse Med. 1989; 18: 1701-1705.

2. Francis, G.S., Goldsmith, S.R., Ziesche, S.M. and Cohn, J.N. Response of plasma norepinephrine and epinephrine to dynamic exercise in patients with congestive heart failure. Am J Cardiol. 1982; 49: 1152-1156.

3. Francis, G.S., Benedict, C., Johnstone, D.E., et al. Comparison of neuroendocrine activation in patients with left ventricular dysfunction with and without congestive heart failure. Circulation. 1990; 82: 1724-1729.

4. Cohn, J.N., Levine, T.B., Olivari, M.T., et al. Plasma norepinephrine as a guide to prognosis in patients with chronic congestive heart failure. N Engl J Med. 1984; 311: 819-824.

5. Swedberg, K., Eneroth, P., Kjekshus, J. and Wilhelmsen, L. Hormones regulating cardiovascular function in patients with severe congestive heart failure and their relation to mortality. Circulation. 1990; 82: 1730-1736.

6. Hasenfuss, G. and Just, H. Clinical relevance of long-term therapy with levodopa and orally active dopamine analogues in patients with chronic congestive heart failure. Basic Res Cardiol. 1989; 84 Suppl 1: 191-196.

7. Francis, G.S., Parks, R. and Cohn, J.N. The effects of bromocriptine in patients with congestive heart failure. Am Heart J. 1983; 106: 100-106.

8. Van Veldhuisen, D.J., Crijns, H.J., Girbes, A.R.J., Tob', T.J.M., Wiesfeld, A.C.P. and Lie, K.I. Electrophysiologic profile of ibopamine in patients with congestive heart failure and ventricular tachycardia and relation to its effects on hemodynamics and plasma catecholamines. Am J Cardiol. 1991; 68: 1194-1202.

9. Rajfer, S.I., Rossen, J.D., Douglas, F.L., Goldberg, L.I. and Karrison, T. Effects of long-term therapy with oral ibopamine on resting hemodynamics and exercise capacity in patients with heart failure: relationship to the generation of N-methyldopamine and to plasma norepinephrine levels. Circulation. 1986; 73: 740-748.

10. Nakano, T., Morimoto, Y., Kakuta, Y., et al. Acute effects of ibopamine hydrochloride on hemodynamics, plasma catecholamine levels, renin activity, aldosterone, metabolism and blood gas in patients with severe congestive heart failure. Arzneimittelforschung. 1986; 36: 1829-1834.

11. Girbes, A.R.J., Van Veldhuisen, D.J., Smit, A.J., Drent-Bremer, A., Meijer, S. and Reitsma, W.D. Renal and neurohumoral effects of ibopamine and metoclopramide in normal man. Br J Clin Pharmacol. 1991; 31: 701-704.

12. Mannelli, M., Pupilli, C., Fabbri, G., et al. Endogenous dopamine (DA) and DA2 receptors: a mechanism limiting excessive sympathetic-adrenal discharge in humans. J Clin Endocrinol Metab. 1988; 66: 626-631.

13. Van Veldhuisen, D.J., Girbes, A.R.J., Van Den Broek, S.A.J. and Lie, K.I. Ibopamine lowers catecholamines during exercise in patients with heart failure. J Am Coll Cardiol. 1991; 17: 353A.

14. Corbalan, R., Jalil, J., Chamorro, G., Casanegra, P. and Valenzuela, P. Effects of captopril versus milrinone therapy in modulating the adrenergic nervous system response to exercise in congestive heart failure. Am J Cardiol. 1990; 65: 644-649.

Role of Plasma Dopamine for Regulation of Blood Pressure in Humans

M. Yoshimura, T. Komori, T. Kimura,
T. Nakanishi and H. Takahashi

Department of Clinical Laboratory and Medicine, Kyoto Prefectural
University of Medicine, Kawaramachi-hirokoji, Kyoto 602, Japan

Key Words: Free dopamine, Sulfoconjugated dopamine,
Blood pressure, Circadian pattern, Exercise, HPLC

ABSTRACT

To examine whether plasma free dopamine (DA) or sulfoconjugated DA plays a role for regulation of blood pressure (BP), we
developed methods to measure free and sulfoconjugated DA levels in
plasma and estimated DA levels during exercise and over a 24 hour
period. Over the 24-hour monitoring periods, plasma sulfoconjugated DA decreased during sleep and increased during awaked state,
while free DA levels did not change. No correlation was observed
between BP and DA levels. During exercise, free DA levels increased at heavy work load accompaning with increased plasma
lactic acid levels. Sulfoconjugated DA levels in response to
exercise exhibited a different pattern from that of free DA level,
and decreased or increased at each individual. A positive correlation was observed between free DA and lactic acid levels, but
not BP. These results suggest that plasma free DA does not regulate BP directly and that sulfoconjugated DA has the buffering
mechanisms to supply or store free DA for physiologic require-
ments.

INTRODUCTION

There are considerable evidences that dopamine (DA) plays an

important role in regulating blood pressure (BP) through a variety

of central and peripheral dopaminergic mechanisms (1-5). DA is

released from the sympathetic neural terminals, adrenal glands as

well as kidneys, and is synthesized from circulating L-DOPA. In the peripheral dopaminergic mechanisms, the released DA is involved in the presynaptic regulation of noradrenaline (NA) release from the sympathetic nerves, the regulation of natriuresis in the kidneys and the modulation of the release of various hormones such as aldosterone.

Abnormalities in these dopaminergic mechanisms are involved in the elevation of BP and the retention of sodium (4.5). The experimental inhibition of DA biosynthesis by carbidopa, the inhibitor of peripheral–DOPA–decarboxylase, accelerates hypertension (HT) in spontaneously hypertensive rats (SHR) exhibiting the diminished natriuresis and the enhanced release of NA from the kidneys (4). In humans, decreased dopaminergic mechanisms appear to be involved in patients with salt–sensitive HT, a subgroup of essential HT (5). These hypertensive patients have reduced DA release from their kidneys as well as a decreased dopaminergic modulation of aldosterone release. These observations suggest that deranged–dopaminergic mechanisms are involved in the pathogenesis of in at least some types of essential HT.

In the present study, we developed methods to measure the free and sulfoconjugated DA levels in plasma and investigated the role of plasma DA in the regulation of BP in humans.

METHODS

Methods for plasma DA measurement

The plasma free catecholamines (CA) concentrations were measured by high–performance liquid chromatography (HPLC, Tosoh Co.) (6). The detection limits of the various CA were 0.01 pmol/ml for adrenaline (A) and 0.03 pmol/ml for NA and DA. For the measurement of total (free plus sulfoconjugated) CA, we used an enzymatic hydrolysis of the sulfoconjugated CA with sulfatase (Sigma) prior to the HPLC analysis.

Reproducibility of free CA measurement in the intraassay

variation was less than 2.2% for both the plasma NA and A and 12.6% for the DA. The intraassay coefficient variation (CV) for the total CA was less than 4.3% for total A, 1.9% for NA and 1.5% for DA.

Plasma DA measurements for 24 hours

Five healthy male volunteers (20–28 years) were remained in a metabolic room in the hospital for 48 hours. After allowing 20 hours for acclimatization to the hospital environments, an intravenous catheter was inserted into an antecubital vein where it remained in place for more than 24 hours. The blood samples for the CA measurements were drawn into an ice chilled tube containing 10 mg of EDTA-2Na at every 30 min intervals from 1730 to 1700 hours. The blood was obtained when the subjects were in a sitting position during the day-time and in a supine position at night during sleep. The BP and heart rate (HR) were measured using an automated sphygmomanometer (Colin).

Plasma DA measurements during exercise

Six healthy male volunteers (20–34 years) without prior exercise training participated in this study. Blood samples for the CA and lactic acid measurements were obtained through an intravenous catheter. The BP and HR were measured using an automated sphygmomanometer. After resting for 30 min, the subjects performed a graded exercise test on a treadmill using Bruce protocol. During rest (in the supine position), exercise (in the standing position) and post exercise (the supine position), the BP, HR, plasma CA and lactic acid levels were monitored. Lactic acid levels were measured using chemical analyzer Ectachem (Kodak).

RESULTS

24-hour plasma DA levels

As shown in Fig. 1, the plasma free DA levels did not exhibited a clear circadian pattern. However, the sulfoconjugated DA levels clearly exhibited a circadian pattern, characterized by higher levels when the subjects were awake and lower levels at night when they were asleep. Both the plasma free and sulfoconjugated NA as well as A concentration showed a circadian pattern. There were large individual variations in the plasma DA levels at each time point and posture. No correlation was observed between the BP and the plasma DA levels.

Exercise and plasma DA levels

The BP and HR increased during the graded exercise. The plasma free NA and A concentrations were increased from the levels recorded during the initial stage of exercise; however the plasma free DA levels began to increase at the time the exercise changed from aerobic to anaerobic (Fig. 2). During exercise, there was a positive correlation between the free DA and lactic acid levels, indicating that free DA might play a significant role in maintaining adequate blood flow to protect against further increases in lactic acid. There was also a positive correlation between the BP and free NA concentration as well as free A but not free DA. A positive correlation was observed between the diastolic BP and sulfoconjugated DA levels. After exercise, the BP, HR, free NA and A levels returned to their basal levels. The plasma free DA levels gradually decreased to basal.

DISCUSSION

HPLC has been used clinically for the measurement of the plasma levels of both free NA and A. However the plasma free DA concentration has been undetectable by HPLC, even when large volumes of plasma are used. A radioenzymatic assay is superior to

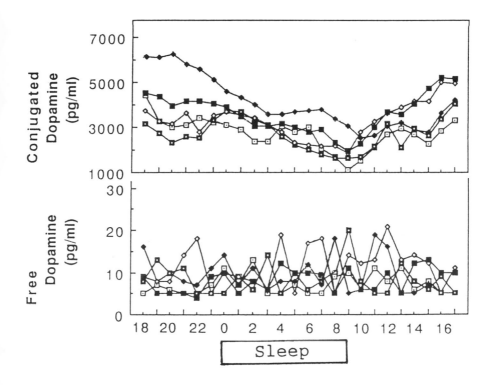

FIG.1 Plasma free and sulfoconjugated dopamine levels in normal subjects throughout a 24-hour period. DA: dopamine.

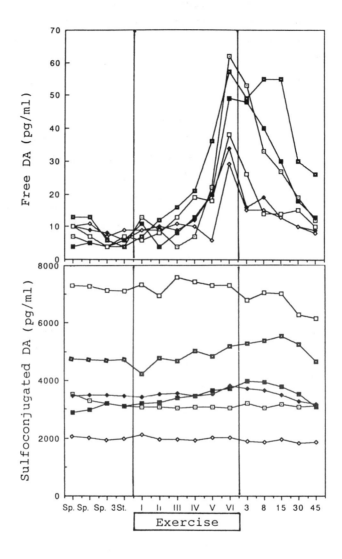

FIG.2 Plasma free and sulfoconjugated dopamine levels during and
after exercise.   Exercise was performed on a treadmill using the
Bruce protocol.   Sp: supine, St: standing, I–VI: exercise stage,
3–45: minutes after exercise.

previous HPLC assays, not only because it is more sensitive but also because less plasma is required for the assay. Nonetheless, because the sensitivity limit of this assay is near the basal level of free DA in the plasma. It is also not well suited for measuring the concentration of free DA in the plasma of normal subjects. With recent technical advances in HPLC, a fully automated HPLC analyzer with an autosampler was developed by Tosoh Co. Ltd Tokyo (6), which is capable of measuring the free CA concentration easily and sensitively without any procedure of extraction. Using both an enzymatic hydrolysis of the conjugated CA and a sensitive HPLC analysis, we have developed a method to simultaneously measure both the free and sulfoconjugated CA levels in human plasma.

The plasma levels of free and conjugated DA in our normal subjects were similar to previously reported values (7). Since the plasma free DA levels in previous studies (7–13) were near the detection limits of the assay, these data were variable. Some studies have reported relatively low free DA concentrations (5–20 pg/ml) in the plasma (7–9). However, other studies found higher levels of free DA (50–140 pg/ml) in the plasma (10–12). These differences in the plasma free DA levels may be due to the detection limits of the CA assay system or to postural effects i.e., changes in the free DA levels as a results of reclining, sitting or standing. Our values for the plasma free DA levels are almost compatible with the former study results (7–9).

The plasma levels of the total (free plus conjugated) DA were also variable (7–12). Since glucuronoconjugated DA is present in minute amounts in human blood (7), the total plasma DA concentration can be regarded as the free plus the sulfoconjugated DA concentrations. We observed wide individual variations in the free and sulfoconjugated DA levels in our study as has been found in previous studies (7–12).

When we measured the plasma DA levels throughout a 24 hour

period, we observed a circadian pattern in the sulfoconjugated, but not in the free DA levels, in daytime sitting and nocturnal reclining position. On the other hand, in daytime and nocturnal recumbent position, there is a report of the circadian pattern of the plasma free DA levels, decreasing during night with sleep and increasing during daytime with awaked state, such as NA and A as are circadian pattern (13).

The plasma DA levels are affected by a number of environmental factors, such as posture, physical activity, diet, stress, mental state, and whether one is asleep or awake as are the plasma levels of NA and A. Higher DA levels in the plasma are observed when one is standing, working and awake than when one is supine, resting or sleeping. These environmental factors may account for the different results of the plasma free DA levels.

During exercise, the BP, HR, lactic acid levels and plasma free CA concentrations increased. The increase in the plasma free DA concentrations accompanied the increase in the lactic acid levels. The pattern of the rise in the free DA concentration was different from those of NA and A, suggesting that the kinetics of free DA use and elimination are different from those of free NA and A.

As for the plasma sulfoconjugated CA concentrations, individual differences were observed during exercise, probably as a result of individual difference in phenolsulfotransferase activity. The plasma sulfoconjugated NA, A and DA concentrations changed during exercise; however, the pattern of change in the sulfoconjugated CA levels in each subject was different from that of the free CA. The circulating free and sulfoconjugated CA levels are influenced by a number of the factors. During exercise, CA is released in large quantities from the sympathetic neuronal terminals and adrenal medulla. This can be utilized for physical works or catabolized by monoamine oxidase (MAO) as well as catechol-o-methyltransferase (COMT) in tissues. It can also circulate in the blood in the free form. Excess free CA can be converted into sulfoconjugated CA and that the sulfoconjugated CA can be converted into free CA when needed. At the maximum work load, the exhaustive subjects had markedly elevated free and decreased sulfoconjugated CA levels. These results suggest that sulfoconjugated CA can be converted into free CA by plasma or tissue sulfatases and that sulfoconjugated CA can serve as a reservoir of CA, from which free CA can be rapidly produced when needed.

After exercise, the plasma free NA and A concentrations decreased rapidly following a decrease with BP and HR. The plasma free DA concentration decreased slowly. There was a difference in the disappearance of kinetics between free NA as well as A and free DA. On the other hand, the plasma sulfoconjugated NA and A levels increased after the end of exercise, indicating an enhanced conversion from free NA and A into sulfoconjugated form. Recent studies (14–16) have suggested a role for conjugation or deconjugation mechanisms in the regulation of the free CA levels. Sulfoconjugated DA can be converted directly into free DA or NA and sulfate in the presence of tissue DA-β –hydroxylase (14–16). When the tissue demand for free CA exceeds the available supply, conjugated CA can be converted into free CA through a deconjugation pathway. Therefore it seems likely that conjugated CA may act as a dynamic regulator of the hemodynamic and metabolic effects of free CA and can serve as a reservoir to supply free CA when needed.

In conclusion, the plasma free DA levels did not correlate with changes in the BP over a 24–hour period and during exercise. These results suggest that the plasma free DA does not regulate BP directly. The mutual convertions between free and sulfoconjugated DA seem to participate the BP regulation. Therefore we believe that the sulfoconjugated DA may serve as a reservoir to supply free NA and DA when needed. However, many questions about the mechanisms involved in this regulation remain unanswered, and more studies are needed to clarify the physiological role of sulfoconjugated DA.

ACKNOWLEDGMENTS

This study was supported in part by a Grant-in Aid for Scientific Research from the Japanese Ministry of Education, Science and Culture.

REFERENCES

1. Taylor, A. A., Fennell, W.H., Feldman, M.B., Brandon, B.S., Gions, J.Z., Mitchell, J.R. Activation of peripheral dopamine presynaptic receptors lowers blood pressure and heart rate in dogs. Hypertension. 1983; 5: 226–234.

2. Lokhandwala, M.F. & Jandhyala, B.S. The role of the nervous system in the vascular actions of dopamine. J Pharmacol Exp Ther. 1979; 210: 120–126.

3. Felder, R.A., Blecher, M., Eisner, G.M., Jose, P.A. Cortical tubular and glomerular dopamine receptors in the kidney. Am J Physiol. 1984; 246: F557–F568.

4. Yoshimura, M., Kambara, S., Takahashi, H., Okabayashi, H., Ijichi, H. Involvement of dopamine in development of hypertension in spontaneously hypertensive rat; effect of carbidopa, inhibitor of peripheral dopa decarboxylase. Clin Exp Hypertens. 1987; A9: 1585–1599

5. Shikuma, R., Yoshimura, M., Kambara, S., Yamazaki, H., Takashina, R., Takahashi, H., Takeda, K., Ijichi, H. Dopaminergic modulation of salt sensitivity in patients with essential hypertension. Life Sci. 1986; 38: 915–921.

6. Iwada, T., Kuroki M., Ohta, K, Ishimura, S., Takahashi H., Watanabe, H. Development of fully automated catecholamine analyzer HLC–8030. J Tosoh Res. 1988; 32: 59–64.

7. Yoneda, S., Alexander, N., Vlachakis, N.D. Enzymatic deconjugation of catecholamines in human and rat plasma and red blood cell lysate. 1983; 33: 935–942.

8. de Champlain, J., Bouvier, M., Cleroux, J., Farley, L. Free

and conjugated catecholamines in plasma and red blood cells of normotensive and hypertensive patients. Clin Exp Hypert. 1984; A6: 523–537.

9. Miura, Y., Takahashi M., Sano, N., Kimura, S., Toriyabe, S., Ishizuka, Y., Noshiro, T., Ohashi, H., Sugawara, T., Watanabe, H., Yoshinaga, K., De Quattro, V. Plasma levels of unconjugated dopamine in various types of hypertension. J Cardiovasc Pharmacol. 1987; 10: S167–A169.

10. Johnson, G.A., Baker, C.A, Smith, R.T. Radioenzymatic assay of sulfate conjugates of catecholamines and dopa in plasma. Life Sci. 1980; 26: 1591–1598.

11. Kuchel, O., Buu, N.T., Hamet, P., Larochelle, P. Catecholamine sulfates and platelet phenolsulfotransferase activity in essential hypertension. J Lab Clin Med. 1984; 104: 238–244.

12. Ratgh, D., Knoll, E., Wisser, H. Plasma free and conjugated catecholamines in clinical disorders. Life Sci. 1986; 39: 557–564.

13. Sowers, J.R., Vlachakis, N.D. Circadian variation in plasma dopamine levels in man. J Endocrinol Invest. 1984; 7: 341–345.

14. Buu, N.T., Kuchel, O. The direct conversion of dopamine 3-0-sulfate to norepinephrine by dopamine- -hydroxylase. Life Sci. 1979; 24: 783–790.

15. Oka, M., Ishimura, Y., Tsunematsu, T., Minaguchi, K., Ohushi, T., Matsumoto, K. Effects of administration of dopamine and L-dopa to dogs on their plasma level of dopamine sulfate. Biochem Pharmacol. 1987; 36: 3205–3208.

16. Huq, A.H.M.M., Matsuoka, S., Karahashi, Y., Kuroda, Y., Mo, S.J., Ohuchi, T., Oka, M. Dopamine 4-sulfate: effects on isolated perfused rat heart and role of atria. Life Sci. 1988; 43: 1599–1606.

A Role for Intrarenal Dopamine in Sodium Homeostasis in Hypertension?

D.F. Schoors and A.G. Dupont

Department of Pharmacology and Hypertension and Clinical
Pharmacology Unit, University Hospital, Free University of
Brussels, 1090 Brussels, Belgium

ABSTRACT

We assessed the effects of low dose dopamine (3 µg/kg/min) on renal function in healthy volunteers, with a special emphasis on lithium clearance and on nephrogenic cAMP formation. In healthy volunteers, dopamine increased renal blood flow and increased urinary sodium excretion. This natriuretic response appears to be due to interaction with proximal tubular dopamine receptors, which are positively coupled to adenylate cyclase. An increased dopamine-induced natriuresis and nephrogenous cAMP formation was observed in hypertensive patients.

In Wistar-Kyoto (WKY) and spontaneously hypertensive rats (SHR) intravenous infusion of fenoldopam (1 µg/kg/min) increased renal blood flow and urinary sodium excretion. The renal tubular response to fenoldopam was enhanced in the WKY after chronic blockade of endogenous dopamine synthesis. A similar exaggerated natriuretic response to fenoldopam was seen in SHR. The natriuretic response to an oral sodium load in the SHR was significantly less pronounced than that observed in the WKY. Chronic blockade of renal dopamine synthesis resulted in an inadequate natriuretic response to oral salt loading in the WKY, mimicking the response obtained in the SHR. This is in agreement with the hypothesis that a deficiency of the intrarenal dopaminergic system (i.e. abnormal renal tubular dopamine synthesis) in the spontaneously hypertensive rat may play a role in the inadequate handling of a sodium load and in the pathogenesis of hypertension in this rat model.

INTRODUCTION

During the last decade, dopamine has been recognized as an important neurotransmitter in the peripheral nervous system (1). The peripheral dopamine receptors are currently subdivided into two pharmacologically distinct subtypes, designated as D1- and D2-receptors (previously called DA1- and DA2- receptors)(2).

The classification is based on pharmacological and biochemical differences and highly selective agonists, antagonists and radioligands of both D1- and D2-receptors and binding-sites have been developed (3). Dopamine itself acts on both, D1- and D2-receptors. The biochemical difference between the two receptor subtypes is based on the opposite control of the adenylate cyclase activity: D1-receptors were reported to be positively coupled to adenylate cyclase, whereas D2-receptors are negatively coupled to this enzyme (4). Peripheral D1-receptors have been characterized on vascular smooth muscle cells of several vascular beds and on proximal tubular cells. Stimulation of these receptors results in respectively, vasodilation and natriuresis (5). D2-receptors are localized presynaptically on sympathetic nerve endings, and stimulation of these receptors results in inhibition of neuronal noradrenaline release (6).

Increasing evidence suggests that the kidney is the main source of urinary dopamine and that this intrarenal dopamine could act as an endogenous natriuretic factor (7-9). Intrarenal dopamine may originate from renal dopaminergic neurons, which have been shown to be present in several species (10). Although some of the intrarenally produced dopamine may originate from specific dopaminergic nerves, it appears that the main source of renal dopamine is the decarboxylation of L-dopa within the proximal tubular cells. Circulating L-dopa is filtered at the glomerulus and then taken up into the proximal tubular cells, where it is converted by dopa decarboxylase to dopamine (11). High concentrations of the enzyme dopa decarboxylase have indeed been found in renal tissue (12). Administration of carbidopa, a dopa-decarboxylase inhibitor, results in a fall in urinary dopamine (13).

Studies, using γ-L-glutamyl-L-dopa (gludopa), have provided further evidence suggesting that endogenous dopamine is formed from L-dopa. Indeed, administration of gludopa, which is converted by g-glutamyl-transferase to dopa and subsequently by dopa-decarboxylase to dopamine, resulted in an about 500-fold increase in urinary dopamine and a significant natriuresis, without any change in plasma dopamine (14). Furthermore, it has been observed in man that renal dopamine production increases in response to a salt load, suggesting that renal dopamine may play a role in sodium handling.

In hypertensive patients a defective ability to excrete a salt load is observed (11,15), and some studies have shown that the urinary dopamine response to salt loading is abnormal in hypertensive patients (16). This may suggest a deficiency of the intrarenal dopaminergic system in hypertension.

The aim of the present work was to gain more information on the site and on the mechanisms of action of the natriuretic effects of dopamine and dopamine receptor agonists, both in man and rats, and also to assess the possibility of a deficiency of the renal dopaminergic system in hypertension.

EXPERIMENTAL DATA

Renal response to dopamine receptor stimulation in healthy young and middle-aged volunteers and in patients with hypertension.

We assessed the effects of low dose intravenous dopamine on renal function in 7 healthy young volunteers (age range from 21 to 24 years), with a special emphasis on nephrogenic cAMP formation. In these healthy volunteers we also monitored glomerular filtration rate and renal plasma flow using a constant IV infusion technique with ^{51}Cr-EDTA and ^{123}I-hippuran. The healthy volunteers were studied a second time after pretreatment with lithium. Lithium clearance can be used as a marker for proximal tubular sodium reabsorption. The dopamine-induced changes in sodium excretion and nephrogenous cAMP were also studied in 9 middle-aged hypertensive patients (34-65 years) and in 6 age-matched normotensive subjects (35-65 years).

The study protocol was the same in the 3 different patient-groups. Dopamine (in a dose of 3 µg/kg/min) was infused during 60 min, preceded and followed by infusion of saline. Timed 20 min urine collections were performed for the determination of sodium (and lithium) and urinary cAMP, whereas mid period blood samples were performed for the determination of sodium, lithium, cAMP and several hormones known to be involved in sodium homeostasis. Blood pressure and heart rate were monitored as well.

During infusion with dopamine there was a progressive increase in renal plasma flow which reached its maximum at the end of the infusion. Lithium per se had no effect on the renal vasodilatory response induced by dopamine. There was no significant change of glomerular filtration rate. Furthermore, during these experiments there was no significant change of blood pressure or heart rate. Plasma renin activity, plasma aldosterone, antidiuretic hormone and atrial natriuretic factor were not significantly changed during the infusion with dopamine. Urinary sodium excretion increased significantly in response to dopamine, and this natriuretic response was not changed by lithium pretreatment. Nephrogenous cAMP formation increased significantly in response to infusion of this low dose of dopamine. The dopamine-induced changes in renal plasma flow did not correlate with the dopamine-induced changes in urinary sodium excretion (r=0.31; ns). However, a significant correlation was found between the increase in urinary sodium excretion and the increase in nephrogenous cAMP (r=0.88; p<0.01), suggesting that dopamine increased urinary sodium excretion through interaction with a adenylate cyclase-linked receptor. Furthermore, the dopamine-induced increase in urinary sodium excretion correlated significantly with the dopamine-induced increase in the fractional excretion of lithium (r=0.94; p<0.01). Therefore, these data suggest that dopamine increases urinary sodium excretion through interaction with a adenylate cyclase-linked receptor, localized at the proximal tubule (17).Others have indeed demonstrated the presence of proximal tubular dopamine receptors (by radioligand and autoradiographic techniques) in animals (18).

The dopamine-induced natriuresis (Figure 1a) and the increase in nephrogenous cAMP formation (Figure 1b) were significantly less pronounced in the middle-aged normotensive subjects when compared to the younger normotensive volunteers.

In hypertensive patients both the dopamine-induced natriuresis (Figure 1a) and the increase in nephrogenous cAMP formation (Figure 1b) were significantly more pronounced than in the age-matched normotensive volunteers (19).

Renal vasodilatory and natriuretic responses to the intravenous infusion of a low dose of fenoldopam, a selective D1-receptor agonist.

In a first series of experiments 12 Wistar-Kyoto rats (WKY) and 12 spontaneously hypertensive rats (SHR) were infused with a low dose of fenoldopam (1 µg/kg/min). In preliminary studies it was shown that this dose of fenoldopam produced a renal vasodilation without a significant effect on systemic hemodynamics. The infusion of fenoldopam during 1 hour was preceded and followed by the infusion of saline. A bladder catheter was inserted to allow timed 30 minutes urine collections for the determination of urinary sodium excretion. Blood pressure and heart rate were monitored continuously, and renal blood flow was measuredusing a electromagnetic flow sensor. In the normotensive rats fenoldopam significantly decreased renal vascular resistance (-27.3%; p<0.05) and the renal vasodilatory response was significantly more pronounced in the SHR (-56.0%; p<0.01). In the WKY a gradual increase in urinary sodium excretion was observed, which reached statistical significance at the end of the infusion (+86.2%; p<0,05); the SHR demonstrated a significantly more pronounced increase in urinary sodium excretion(176.6%; p<0.01).

In a second series of experiments we pretreated two other groups of 12 WKY and 12 SHR with carbidopa (100 mg/kg of food for 10 days) in order to block endogenous dopamine synthesis. Thereafter they were again infused with fenoldopam following the same protocol as in the first series of experiments. Pretreatment with carbidopa did not influence the renal vasodilator response of fenoldopam in the WKY (-25.3%; p<0.05), and this observation may suggest that renal tubular dopamine is not involved in the control of renal vascular dopamine receptors. In the WKY, pretreatment with carbidopa significantly increased the natriuretic effect of fenoldopam (172.6%; p<0.01), resulting in a similar response as in the SHR. In the SHR pretreatment with carbidopa had no effect on the natriuretic effect of fenoldopam (174.0%; p<0.01).

In a third line of experiments the effect of age on the renal response to D1-receptor stimulation was studied. Six 3 month old, six 6 month old and six 12 month old WKY were infused with fenoldopam again using a similar protocol as the one described earlier. The renal vasodilatory response to fenoldopam was similar in the 3 different age groups, although the oldest rats showed a slightly but not significant lower response to fenoldopam.However, the natriuretic response of the youngest rats (+86.2%) was significantly more pronounced than the one observed in 6 month old rats (+68.5%), which in turn was larger than the one obtained in the oldest rats (+49.0%), indicating a reduction of the natriuretic response to fenoldopam with increasing age.

The results of these experiments show that D1-receptor stimulation results in an increased renal blood flow and an increased urinary sodium excretion, both in normotensive and spontaneously hypertensive rats. In the SHR an enhanced fenoldopam-induced natriuresis

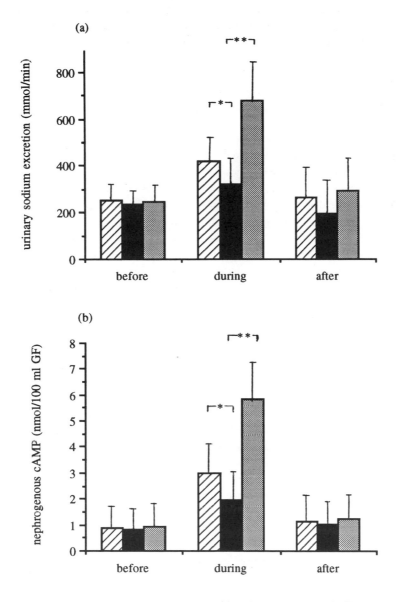

FIG 1. Response of urinary sodium excretion (a) and nephrogenous cAMP formation (b) to infusion of dopamine (3 µg/kg/min) in young normotensive subjects (hatched bar)(n=7), in middle-aged normotensive subjects (closed bar)(n=6) and in hypertensive patients (spotted bar)(n=9). Values are means ± SD; *p<0.05, **p<0.01, significant differences as compared to the response obtained in middle-aged normotensive subjects.

is found and this response can be mimicked in the WKY when its endogenous dopamine production is blocked by carbidopa. With increasing age a diminished natriuretic response to low-dose fenoldopam is found

Renal dopamine response to sodium loading in both normotensive Wistar-Kyoto and spontaneously hypertensive rats.

In a first line of experiments we studied 12 WKY and 12 SHR, which were housed in individual metabolic cages. They received a normal sodium-containing diet (24 mmol of Na per kg of food) for 10 days and then from day 10 till day 17 a supplement of 376 mmol of Na per kg of food was added. Daily 24h urine collections were performed to measure urinary sodium and dopamine excretion (HPLC). Blood pressure (tail cuff method) and body weight were monitored on alternate days.

Salt loading resulted in an increase in urinary sodium excretion in both groups of rats, but this increase in urinary sodium excretion was significantly lower. in the SHR, indicating a defective ability to excrete a salt load in the SHR (Figure 2). The WKY demonstrated a significant increase in urinary dopamine excretion upon salt loading (from 10.5 ± 1.7 to 50.3 ± 8.6 µg/day; $p<0.001$), whereas in the SHR no dopamine response was seen. In order to evaluate the role of renal dopamine production in mediating the natriuretic response to oral sodium loading, we also examined the effect of blockade of intrarenal dopamine synthesis on the natriuretic and renal dopamine response to sodium loading.

Therefore, in a second line of experiments we studied 2 additional groups of 12 WKY and 12 SHR, which were pretreated with carbidopa (100 mg/kg of food for 10 days). They were again housed in individual metabolic cages. Salt loading was performed following the same protocol as described earlier. The urinary sodium excretion upon salt loading in WKY was significantly lower when endogenous dopamine was blocked with carbidopa, and was now of the same magnitude as the natriuretic response obtained in SHR (Figure 2). Carbidopa pretreatment did not influence the renal response to a salt load in the SHR (Figure 2). Urinary dopamine was lower in carbidopa-treated WKY, indicating a blockade of endogenous dopamine synthesis. In the carbidopa-treated WKY no response of urinary dopamine was seen upon salt loading, and, similarly, a dopamine response to salt loading was absent in both untreated SHR and carbidopa-treated SHR. Blood pressure was not affected by salt loading in the untreated WKY. Carbidopa slightly increased blood pressure in the WKY and resulted in an increase in blood pressure upon salt loading (+9 mmHg). In both untreated and carbidopa-treated SHR an increase in blood pressure was noted upon salt loading (+13 mmHg).

CONCLUSION

In humans a decreased natriuretic response to low dose dopamine infusion, paralled by a reduced formation of nephrogenous cAMP is found with increasing age. Moreover,

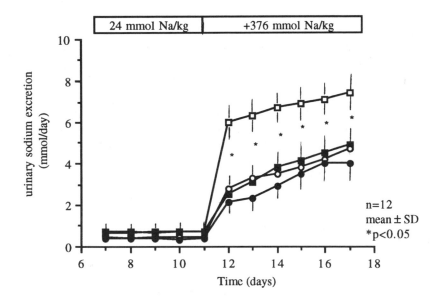

FIG 2. Response of urinary sodium excretion to oral salt load in both untreated (□) and carbidopa-treated WKY (▉) and both untreated (o) and carbidopa-treated SHR (●). Values are means ± SD; n=12 in each group; *p<0.05 significant difference as compared to the normotensive Wistar-Kyoto rat.

we have previously reported that aging is associated with a progressive reduction in urinary dopamine excretion (20). In rats, a decreased natriuretic response to D1-receptor stimulation is observed. Preliminary data also indicate that in rats increasing age is associated with a decrease in urinary dopamine excretion (unpublished observation). This may suggest that aging is associated with a progressive reduction of the renal dopaminergic tone, which is characterized by a decreased renal dopamine formation, and a reduced response to exogenous D1-receptor stimulation, due to either a decrease in receptor number and/or a reduced receptor-effector coupling.

In patients with hypertension an enhanced natriuretic response and nephrogenous cAMP formation to exogenous dopamine is observed. In our rat studies, we observed an increased natriuretic response to D1-receptor stimulation in the SHR; this response can be mimicked in WKY by blockade of endogenous dopamine synthesis. Furthermore, we observed a reduced natriuretic response to a salt load in the SHR with a lack of the normal dopamine response, and also this abnormal response can be reproduced in the WKY by blockade of its endogenous dopamine synthesis.

It is therefore tempting to hypothesize that hypertension is characterized by a failure of the renal dopaminergic system, which may play a role in the reduced ability to excrete a salt load and in the enhanced sensitivity to exogenous D1-receptor stimulation found both in man and animals with hypertension.

REFERENCES

1. Bell, C., Mann, R. Identification of dopaminergic nerves in humans. Am J Hypertens 1990; 3: 4S-6S.

2. Watson, S., Abbott A. Receptor nomenclature supplement. TiPS 1991: 11.

3. Seeman, P., Grigoriadis, D. Dopamine receptors in brain and periphery. Neurochem Int 1987; 10: 1-25.

4. Stoof, J.C., Kebabian, J.W. Two dopamine receptors: biochemistry, physiology and pharmacology. Life Sci 1984; 35: 2281-2296.

5. Goldberg, L.I., Volkman, P.H., Kohli, J.D. A comparison of the vascular dopamine receptor with other dopamine receptors. Ann Rev Pharmacol Toxicol 1978; 18: 57-79.

6. Dupont, A.G., Lefebvre, R.A., Bogaert, M.G. Identification and characterization of peripheral neuronal dopamine receptors in the rat. Clin Exp Hypertens [A] 1987; 9: 913-929.

7. Kuchel, O., Buu, N.T., Unger, T. Dopamine-sodium relationship: is dopamine a part of the endogenous natriuretic system? Contr Nephrol 1978; 13: 27-36.

8. Lee, M.R. Dopamine, the kidney and essential hypertension: studies with gludopa. Clin Exp Hypertens [A] 1987; 9: 977-986.

9. Bell, C. Endogenous renal dopamine and control of blood pressure. Clin Exp Hypertens [A] 1987; 9: 955-975.

10. Bell, C., Bhathal, P.S., Mann, R., Ryan, G.B. Evidence that dopaminergic sympathetic axons supply the medullary arterioles of human kidney. Histochemistry 1989; 91: 361-364.

11. Lee, M.R. Dopamine and the kidney. Clin Sci 1982; 62: 439-448.

12. Goldstein, M., Fuxe, K., Hokfelt, T. Characterization and tissue localization of catecholamine synthesizing enzymes. Pharmacol Rev 1972; 24: 293-315.

13. Brown, M.J., Dollery, C.T. A specific radioenzymatic assay for dihydroxyphenylalanine (dopa). Plasma dopa may be the precursor of urine free dopamine. Br J clin Pharmac 1981; 11: 79-83.

14. Jeffrey, R.F., MacDonald, T.M., Brown, J., Rae, P.W.H., Lee, M.R. The effect of lithium on the renal response to the dopamine prodrug gludopa in normal man. Br J clin Pharmac 1988; 25: 725-732.

15. Bell, C. Dopamine and the kidney. In: Amenta F, ed. Peripheral dopamine pathophysiology. Boca Raton: CRC Press Inc., 1990: 87-98.

16. Harvey, J.N., Casson, I.F., Clayden, A.D., Cope, G.F., Perkins, C.M., Lee, M.R. A paradoxical fall in urine dopamine output when patients with essential hypertension are given added dietary salt. Clin Sci 1984; 67: 83-88.

17. Schoors, D.F., Dupont, A.G. Further studies on the mechanism of the natriuretic response to low-dose dopamine in man: effect on lithium clearance and nephrogenic cAMP formation. Eur J clin Invest 1990; 20: 385-391.

18. Hedge, S.S., Jadhav, A.L., Lokhandwala, M.F. Role of kidney dopamine in the natriuretic response to volume expansion in rats. Hypertension 1989; 13: 828-834.

19. Schoors, D.F., Dupont, A.G. Increased dopamine-induced nephrogenous cAMP formation in hypertension. Am J Hypertens 1991; 4: 494-499.

20. Gerlo, E.A.M., Schoors, D.F., Dupont, A.G. Age- and sex-related differences for the urinary excretion of norepinephrine, epinephrine and dopamine in adults. Clin Chem 1991; 37: 875-878.

Impairment of Renal Dopamine Receptor Function in Spontaneously Hypertensive Rats

Changjian Chen and Mustafa F. Lokhandwala

Department of Pharmacology, University of Houston, Houston,
Texas, TX 77204-5515, USA

Key Words: Dopamine, DA-1 receptor, Hypertension, Renal Function.

ABSTRACT

Since endogenous dopamine (DA) plays an important role in maintaining body fluid and volume homeostasis, it is proposed that mulfunction of renal DA-ergic system may contribute to certain pathological conditions characterized by impaired renal sodium excretion. Increasing evidence suggests that there is an impaired DA receptor function in spontaneously hypertensive rats (SHR), one of the most studied genetic models of hypertension. We have shown that when subjected to acute volume expansion, adult SHR has diminished endogenous kidney DA-mediated natriuresis and diuresis compared with their WKY counterparts, although urinary DA excretion was increased to a similar degree in both groups. Impaired renal DA receptor function in the SHR was also suggested by the findings that the natriuretic response to DA and DA-1 receptor agonist fenoldopam was reduced in hypertensive animals. It is known that DA-1 receptors in the renal proximal tubule are coupled to both adenylate cyclase and phospholipase C. DA-1 receptor mediated activation of adenylate cyclase is shown to be linked to inhibition of Na^+,H^+-exchanger's activity in the renal proximal tubule. It is reported that DA-1 receptor adenylate cyclase coupling is defective in the renal proximal tubule of SHR, which could contribute to diminished DA-induced inhibition of Na^+,H^+-exchanger's activity in the proximal tubule recently found in these hypertensive rats. We examined the DA-1 receptor phospholipase C coupling process and found that DA-induced activation of phospholipase C is diminished in the SHR. Since protein kinase C activation presumably following DA-1 receptor mediated stimulation of phospholipase C is involved in DA-induced inhibition of Na^+,K^+-ATPase activity, we examined possible change in DA-induced inhibition of Na^+,K^+-ATPase using the basolateral membrane of renal proximal tubule. We found that DA-induced inhibition of Na^+,K^+-ATPase is abolished in the SHR. These observations together suggest that there is an impaired renal DA receptor function in the SHR, which may have pathogenic significance in terms of development as well as maintenance of high blood pressure in this model of hypertension.

Please send all correspondence to:

Mustafa F. Lokhandwala, Ph.D.
Department of Pharmacology
University of Houston
Houston, Texas 77204-5515
Phone: (713) 743-1253
Fax: (713) 743-1259

Introduction

Accumulating evidence suggests that endogenous kidney dopamine (DA) has an important role in regulation of renal sodium excretion (1,2). Both clinical and animal studies have demonstrated that urinary DA excretion is closely correlated with urinary sodium exretion and / or sodium intake. DA receptor blockade as well as inhibition of peripheral DA synthesis by carbidopa leads to attenuation of diuresis and natriuresis induced by sodium loading (1,3,4). In conscious dogs, dose-related antidiuresis and antinatriuresis were observed with intrarenal arterial infusion of selective DA-1 receptor antagonist SCH 23390 (5).

Although the exact mechanisms for the development and maintenance of high blood pressure in genetic hypertension reamin to be elucidated, there is a body of evidence for the primary abnormality within the kidney in the hypertensive process (6,7). Firstly, spontaneously hypertensive rats (SHR) retain sodium avidly prior to the development of hypertension (8,9). Secondly, the blood pressure of the recipient follows that of the donor after cross kidney transplantation between the hypertensives and normotensives in several animal models including SHR (6,10). Furthermore, dietary sodium restriction retards or ameliorates, whereas high sodium diet accelerates or aggravates the hypertensive process as shown both in clinical and animal studies (6,7,11).

There appear to be several renal hormonal mechanisms, alterations of which may be responsible for an abnormal renal handling of sodium in some models of hypertension including SHR (12). Based on the increasing evidence suggesting that renal dopaminergic system is actively involved in regulation of renal sodium excretion (1,2,13,14), it has been suspected that a malfunction of renal DA-ergic system might be present in this type of hypertension, which contributes to the abnormal renal sodium excretion (15,16). In this paper, we present recent findings on the functional changes in renal DA receptor coupled cellular signaling mechanisms in the SHR.

Renal Dopamine and Dopamine Receptor

The functional role of DA as a precursor for norepinephrine and epinephrine and a neurotransmitter in the central nervous system has been known for a long time. However, the importance of DA generated in the kidney in maintaining body fluid and volume homeostais is only recently beginning to be appreciated (1,2). It is well demonstrated that all components necessary to synthesize DA and mediate DA-induced effects are present in various parts of kidneys. The enzyme, dopa-decarboxylase, whch converts L-dopa to DA, is present in abundance in proximal and distal tubules (17,18). The substrate L-dopa is filtered freely from glomerulus and is actively transported into the proximal tubule. Both subtypes of dopamine receptors (DA-1 and DA-2) are present in various parts of the nephron as shown using autoradiography and receptor ligand binding techniques (1,2). DA-1 binding sites have been identified in the main renal vasculature on the muscular layers of the main renal artery and the afferent arterioles (18). DA-2 binding sites are also present in the adventitial and endothelial layers of these vessels, where it is believed that the renal nerve terminals are located (19). DA-1 binding sites are also shown in cultured mesangial cells, although their functional implication, if any, is not known (20). DA-1 and DA-2 receptors are present in the proximal tubule (1,2,21). DA-1 receptors are also present in the cortical collecting duct and medullary thick ascending limb. Specific DA-1 receptor binding sites are also present in other segments of the nephron, although in much smaller quantities. A novel DA-2 receptor named the DA-2k has also been described in inner medullary collecting duct cells, which may also be involved in mediating the DA-induced renal effects (22,23).

Cellular Mechanisms for DA-induced Renal Response

DA promotes renal sodium excretion via several mechanisms. DA-induced renal vasodilation (subsequent increase in renal blood flow and glomerular filtration rate) is mediated mainly by activation of DA-1 receptor located on vascular smooth muscle and partly by activation of presynaptic DA-2 receptor (1,2). Decrease in renal nerve activity mediated by activation of DA-2

C. Chen and M.F. Lokhandwala

receptor located in nerve terminals may also contribute to DA-induced natriuresis. Direct inhibition of tubular sodium transport, which is mediated predominantly by activation of DA-1 receptor located on proximal tubule, is believed to be one of the major mechanisms for endogenous kidney DA and exogenous DA and / or DA receptor agonists induced natriuresis (1,3). The cellular mechanisms mediating DA-induced renal effects are increasingly recognized recently. Similar to central D-1 receptors, peripheral DA-1 receptor is also shown to be positively coupled to adenylate cyclase in renal proximal and cortical collecting tubules as well as in renal vasculature (1,2,24,25), whereas DA-2 receptor is shown to be negatively coupled to adenylate cyclase in renal proximal tubule (26). DA-sensitive cyclic AMP generating system is also described in cultures of rat glomerular mesangial cells (19). In renal proximal tubule, DA-1 receptor is also demonstrated to be coupled to phospholipase C (27,28). Increasing evidence suggests that endogenous kidney DA acts as an intrarenal natriuretic hormone primarily via activation of DA-1 receptors. Activation of adenylate cyclase following occupation of DA-1 receptor is linked to an inhibition of Na^+,H^+-exchanger's activity located in the brush border membrane of renal proximal tubule (29) and an inhibition of Na^+,K^+-ATPase activity in the cortical collecting duct (30). In the medullary thick ascending limb of Henle, DA induced inhibition of Na^+,K^+-ATPase activity is proposed to be due to DA-1 receptor-mediated activation of adenylate cyclase, which produces accumulation of cAMP and the phosphoprotein, DARPP-32(31,32). Although DA is constantly shown to inhibit Na^+,K^+-ATPase in the proximal tubule, the subtype of DA receptor involved in this phenomenon is still arguable. It is proposed by Bertorello and Aperia that DA-induced inhibition of Na^+,K^+-ATPase in the renal proximal tubule involves simultaneous activation of DA-1 and DA-2 receptors (33). Recently we and other have demonstrated that only DA-1 receptor activation is involved in the DA-induced inhibition of Na^+,K^+-ATPase in rat renal proximal tubule (34-36). Protein kinase C is clearly shown to be involved in DA-induced inhibition of Na^+,K^+-ATPase in the proximal tubule (37). We recently found that phospholipase C activation is related to DA-induced inhibition of Na^+,K^+-ATPase activity in the renal proximal tubule suspension, since DA-induced inhibition of Na,K-ATPase in this preparation was abolished in the presence of phospholipase C inhibitor U

73122 (unpublished observation). Therefore it is likely that PKC activation may be an intermediate step linking DA-1 receptor-coupled phospholipase C activation to an inhibition of Na^+,K^+-ATPase activity (1). Interestingly, recently we observed that the basal phospholipase C activity was significantly elevated in renal cortex of rats on high salt diet as compared with those on normal sodium intake, and this increased phospholipase C activity in rats on high salt diet was reduced to control levels by pretreatment of rats with selective DA-1 receptor antagonist SCH 23390 (38). This observation suggests that during acute increase in salt intake, there is an increased production of intrarenal DA which increases phospholipase C activity via stimulation of DA-1 receptors, which in turn would inhibit renal tubular reabsorption possibly via an inhibition of Na^+,K^+-ATPase activity. A novel DA-2k receptor, which is recently demonstrated in the inner medullary collecting duct, could be related to DA-induced release of prostaglandin E2 in these cells and therefore contribute to DA-induced diuresis and natriuresis (22).

Evidence for Impaired Renal DA Receptor Function in SHR

Enhanced urinary DA excretion (39) and increased peripheral DA content in adrenal glands as well as kidneys (40,41) was observed at several developmental stages in SHR. Although endogenous kidney DA synthesis and/or secretion is normal or even increased, there is evidence showing that endogenous kidney DA-mediated natriuresis is diminished in the SHR (15,39).

Earlier studies showed that although kidney DA content and urinary DA excretion were markedly elevated in young SHR, renal sodium excretion was paradoxically less in SHR than their WKY counterparts (39). We have recently observed that urinary DA excretion under basal condition in adult SHR was twice as high as in the age-matched WKY rats, yet there were no differences in basal urinary sodium excretion or urine output (42). When subjected to acute volume loading (5% body weight), the adult SHR demonstrate diminished natriuresis and diuresis, which is related to impaired renal tubular DA receptor function (42). Although diminished DA-mediated diuresis and natriuresis in the SHR could also be attributed to enhanced antinatriuretic forces previously shown in this model, e.g.; enhanced renin angiotensin activity, elevated renal nerve activity (43), there is evidence which suggests an impaired renal DA receptor function in SHR as a causative factor for this phenomenon. It is demonstrated that the volume expansion evoked a similar increase in urinary DA excretion between SHR and WKY groups and selective DA-1 receptor antagonist SCH 23390 significantly attenuated volume expansion-induced natriuresis and diuresis in the normotensive WKY rats, but not in the SHR (42). These observations indicate that inasmuch as endogenous kidney DA synthesis /secretion in the SHR in response to sodium loading is normal or enhanced, diminished endogenous DA-mediated natriuresis therefore involves most likely an impairment of DA receptor function. Further evidence which supports this proposal comes from studies with exogenous DA and DA receptor agonists. Similar to the findings of Felder et al (44), we have also discovered that exogenous administration of DA or the selective DA-1 receptor agonist fenoldopam in a dose which does not produce detectable changes in hemodynamic parameters causes natriuresis and diuresis both in SHR and WKY. However, the magnitude of diuretic and natriuretic response is significantly diminished in SHR compared to WKY rats (42,45).

Defective Renal DA Receptor Coupled Signalling Mechanisms as the Cause for Diminished Renal DA-ergic Function in SHR

Dopamine causes natriuresis predominantly via activation of tubular DA-1 receptor, which is coupled to both adenylate cyclase and phospholipase-C. There is evidence indicating that both of these DA-1 receptor coupled cellular signalling mechanisms are involved in the overall DA-induced natriuresis (1,3,15). Therefore, it is reasonable to hypothesize that a defect in either one or both of these signal transduction pathways might contribute to the diminished natriuretic response to both DA and selective DA-1 receptor agonists seen in the SHR.

The observation that urinary excretion of cyclic AMP was lower in SHR than in WKY rats in spite of elevated urinary DA excretion in SHR suggests a deficiency in the ability of DA to stimulate cyclic AMP production via DA-1 receptor activation (16). Further evidence came from studies showing that DA-1 receptor agonists fenoldopam, SK&F 38393 and SND 911C12, stimulated adenylate cyclase activity of renal proximal tubule to a lesser extent in SHR than in WKY rats (46). It was also demonstrated in these studies that the dissociation constant, maximum receptor density and DA-1 receptor antagonist inhibition constant were similar in SHR and WKY rats (46). These findings together with observation that GTP and Gpp (NH)p enhanced the ability of DA-1 receptor agonists to stimulate adenylate cyclase activity in WKY rats but not in SHR, suggest a defect in the DA-1 receptor second messenger coupling mechanism in the proximal tubule of SHR (46). Recent reports suggest that the defective DA-1 receptor-adenylate cyclase coupling in the renal proximal tubule may contribute to the diminished DA-induced inhibition of Na^+-H^+-exchanger's activity and therefore may be related to enhanced Na^+-H^+ antiport activity observed in renal brush border membrane of SHR (47). There are yet no reports concerning the functional status of DA-1 receptor-adenylate cyclase coupling in other segments of nephron.

We recently have examined the DA-1 receptor phospholipase C coupling in the SHR. It was found that DA-induced activation of phospholipase-C as expressed in terms of fractional release of inositol phosphates was significantly diminished in renal cortical slices of adult SHR as compared to the WKY rats (45). It appears that the diminished DA-induced activation of phospholipase-C in the SHR was due almost entirely to an impaired DA-1 receptor function, since the selective DA-1 receptor antagonist SCH 23390, which blocked 50% of DA-stimulated inositol phosphates production in the WKY rats, did not have any significant effect on DA-induced inositol phosphates production in the SHR (45). We also observed that the basal level of phospholipase-C activity was significantly higher in the SHR than WKY rats. The higher levels of phospholipase C activity in the SHR could be due to enhanced α-adrenoceptor stimulation resulting from elevated renal nerve activity and/or increased peripheral DA production.

Since protein kinase C activation is shown to be involved in DA-induced inhbition of Na^+,K^+-ATPase activity and protein kinase C activation is known to occur following activation of phospholipase C, diminished DA-induced activation of phospholipase C could lead to reduced DA-induced inhibition of Na^+,K^+-ATPase activity. To determine this possibility, we performed experiments in which DA-induced inhibition of Na^+,K^+-ATPase was compared between SHR and

WKY rats using basolateral membrane preparation of renal proximal tubule. DA produced a concentration-related inhibition of Na^+,K^+-ATPase in WKY rats, but not in SHR (48). In addition, DA-induced inhibition of Na^+,K^+-ATPase in WKY rats was antagonized by selective DA-1 receptor antagonist SCH 23390 in a concentration-dependent manner, indicating the involvement of tubular DA-1 receptor in this response (48).

Taken together, all of the experimental evidence suggests that in the SHR there is a defect in renal DA-ergic system which involves the DA-1 receptor-coupled signal transduction pathways, but not renal DA synthesis/secretion. Both DA-1 receptor adenylate cyclase and DA-1 receptor phospholipase-C coupling processes are less efficient in the proximal tubules of adult SHR. Although available evidence does not allow to differentiate whether a defect in these signal transduction pathways is a consequence of sustained hypertension or a fundamental abnormality, it is interesting to note that a defect in tubular DA-1 receptor adenylate cyclase coupling has been shown to be present in young SHR of prehypertensive stage (49), suggesting its pathogenic significance in initiation of hypertensive process in this animal model of hypertension.

Summary

Recent studies show that there is diminished involvement of endogenous kidney DA in regulation of renal sodium excretion in SHR, which may be due to defective DA-ergic signal transduction pathways in renal proximal tubules. The functional significance of impaired renal DA-1 receptor function in terms of its impact on pathophysiological processes in genetic models of hypertension remains to be further determined.

References

1.   Lokhandwala, M.F. & Amenta, F.: Anatomical distribution and function of dopamine receptors in the kidney. FASEB J, 1991, 5: 3023-3030.

2.   Jose, P. A., Raymond, J. R., Bates, M. D., Aperia, A., Felder, R. A. & Carey, R. M.: The renal dopamine receptors. J. Am. Soc. Nephrol. 1992; 2: 1265-1278.

3.   Lokhandwala, M.F. & Hegde, S.S.: Cardiovascular dopamine receptors: role of dopamine and dopamine receptors in sodium excretion. Pharmacol. Toxicol. 1990, 66: 237- 243.

4.   Hegde, S.S., Jadhav, A.L. & Lokhandwala, M.F.: Role of kidney dopamine in the natriuretic response to volume expansion in rats. Hypertension. 1989, 13: 828-834.

5.   Siragy, H. M., Felder, R. A., Howell, N. L., Chevalier, R. L., Peach, M. J. and Carey, R. M.: Evidence that intrarenal dopamine acts as a paracrine substance at the renal tubule. Amer. J. Physiol., 1989; 257: F469-477.

6.   De Wardener, H.E.: The primary role of the kidney and salt intake in the aetiology of essential hypertension. Clin. Sci. 1990a, 79: 193-200.

7.   De Wardener, H.E.: The primary role of the kidney and salt intake in the aetiology of essential hypertension. Clin. Sci. 1990b, 79: 289-297.

8.   Beierwaltes, W.H., Arendshorst, W.J. & Klemmer, P.H.: Electrolyte and water balance in young spontaneously hypertensive rats. Hypertension. 1982, 4:908-915.

9.   Arendshorst, W.J. & Beierwaltes, W.H: Renal tubular reabsorption in spontaneously hypertensive rats. Amer. J. Physiol. 1979, 237:F38-F47.

10.   Rettig, R., Folberth, C., Stauss, H., Kopf, D., Waldherr, R. & Unger, T: Role of the kidney in primary hypertension: a renal transplantation study in rats. Amer. J. Physiol. 1990, 258: F606-F611.

11.   Toal, C.B. & Leenen, F.H.H: Dietary sodium restriction and development of hypertension in spontaneously hypertensive rats. Amer. J. Physiol. 1983, 245: H1081 - H1084.

12.   Carretero, O.A. & Scicli, A.G.: Local hormonal factors (intracrine, autocrine, and paracrine) in hypertension. Hypertension. 1991, 18 (Suppl. I): I-58 - I-69.

13.   Ball, S.G., Oats, H.S. & Lee, M.R: Urinary dopamine in man and rat: effect of inorganic salts on dopamine excretion. Clin. Sci. & Mol. Med. 1978, 55: 167-173.

14.   Carey, R.M., Siragy, H.M. & Felder, R.A.: Physiological modulation of renal function by the renal dopaminergic system. J. Auton. Pharmacol. 1990, 10 (Suppl. 1) :47S-51S.

15.   Chen, C. J. & Lokhandwala, M. F.: Dopaminergic receptors in hypertension. Pharmacology & Toxicology. 1992, 70 (suppl. I): 17-22.

16.   Yoshimura, M., Ikegaki, I., Nishimura, M. & Takahashi, H.: Role of dopaminergic mechanisms in the kidneys for the pathogenesis of hypertension. J. Auto. Pharmacol. 1990, 10 (Suppl. 1): 67S - 72S.

17.   Baines, A.D. & Chan, W.: Production of urine free dopamine from DOPA: a micropuncture study. Life Sci. 1980, 26:253-259.

18.   Zimlichman, R., Levinson, P.P., Kelly, G., Stull, R., Keiser, H.R. & Goldstein, D.S.: Decivation of urinary dopamine from plasma dopa. Clin. Sci. 1988,75: 515-520.

19.   Amenta, F.: Biochemistry and autoradiography of peripheral dopamine receptors. In: Peripheral Dopamine Pathophysiology (Amenta, F., ed) CRC Press, Boca Raton, Florida., 1990, pp: 39-49.

20.   Schultz, P.J., Sedor, J.R. & Abbound, H.F.: Dopaminergic stimulation of cAMP accumulation in cultured rat mesangial cells. Amer. J. Physiol. 1987, 253: H358-364.

21.   Felder, C.C., McKelvey, A.M., Gitler, M.S., Eisner, G.M. & Jose, P.A.: Dopamine receptor subtypes in renal brush border and basolateral membrane. Kidney Int. 1989a, 36: 183-193.

22.   Huo, T & Healy, D. P.: (3H) domperidone binding to the kidney inner medullary collecting duct dopamine-2k (DA2k) receptor. J. Pharmacol. Exp. Ther. 1991, 258: 424-428.

23.   Huo, T & Healy, D. P.: Characterization of dopamine-2k (DA2k) receptor in the kidney inner medulla. Proc Natl Acad Sci USA, 1991, 88: 3170-3174.

24.   Baldi, E., Pupilli, C., Amenta, F. & Mannelli, M.: Presence of dopamine-dependent adenylate cyclase activity in human renal cortex. Eur. J. Pharmacol. 1988, 149: 351-356.

25.   Felder, R.A., Albrecht, F., Eisner, G.M. & Jose, P.A.: The signal transducer for the dopamine-regulated sodium transport in renal cortical brush border membrane vesicles. Amer. J. Hypertension. 1990a, 3: 47S-50S.

26.   Ricci, A., Collier, W. L., Rossodivita, I. and Amenta, F.: Dopamine receptors mediating inhibition of the cyclic adenosine monophosphate generating system in the rat renal cortex. J. Auton. Pharmacol., 11:121-128, 1991.

27.   Felder, C.C., Blecher, M. & Jose, P.A.: Dopamine-1 mediated stimulation of phospholipase-C activity in rat renal cortical membranes. J. Biol. Chem. 1989b, 2674: 8739-8745.

28.   Vyas, S.J., Eichberg, J. & Lokhandwala, M.F.: Characterization of receptors involved in dopamine induced activation of phospholipase-C in rat renal cortex. J. Pharmacol. Exp. Ther. 1992, 260: 134-139.

29.   Felder, C.C., Campbell, T., Albrecht, F. and Jose, P.A.: Dopamine inhibits Na^+-H^+exchanger activity in renal BBMV by stimulation of adenylate cyclase. Am. J. Physiol. 259: F297-303, 1990.

30.   Satoh, T., Cohen, H.T. & Katz, A. I.: Intracellular signaling in the regulation of renal Na^+,K^+-ATPase. 1. role of cyclic AMP and phospholipase A2. J. Clin. Invest. 1992, 89: 1496-1500.

31.   Aperia, A; Fryckstedt, J; Svensson, L; Hemmings, JC. Jr; Nairn, AC; Greengard, P: Phosphorylated Mr 32,000 dopamine- and cAMP-regulated phosphoprotein inhibits Na^+,K^+-ATPase activity in renal tubule cells. Proc. Natl. Acad. Sci. USA. 1991; 88:2798-2801.

32.   Fryckstedt, J., Meister, B. & Aperia, A.: Control of electrolyte transport in the kidney through a dopamine- and cAMP-regulated phosphoprotein, DARPP-32. J. Auton. Pharmacol. 1992, 12: 183-189.

33.   Bertorello, A. and Aperia, A.: Inhibition of proximal tubule Na^+,K^+-ATPase activity requires simultaneous activation of DA1 and DA2 receptors. Amer. J. Physiol. 259: F924-928, 1990.

34.   Chen, C.J. & Lokhandwala, M.F.: Dopamine inhibits in rat renal proximal tubule via DA-1 receptor activation. J. Pharmacol. Exp. Ther. (submitted).

35.   Seri, I., Kone, B. C., Gullans, S. R., Brenner, B. M. and Ballermann, B. J.: Inhibition of Na^+,K^+-ATPase (Na-K) in rat renal cortical tubule cells (RCTC) by locally formed DA (DA) involves DA-1 but not DA-2 receptors. Kidney Int., 35:320, 1989 (Abstract).

36.   Baines, A.D., Ho, P. & Drangova, R.: Proximal tubular dopamine production regulates basolateral Na^+-K^+-ATPase. Amer. J. Physiol. 1992, 262: F566 - 571.

37.   Bertorello, A. and Aperia, A.: Na^+-K^+-ATPase is an effector protein for protein kinase C in renal proximal tubule cells. Am. J. Physiol., 256:F370-373, 1989.

38.   Vyas, S.J., Jadhav, A.L., Eichberg, J. & Lokhandwala, M.F.: Dopamine receptor-mediated activation of phospholipase C is associated with natriuresis during high salt intake. Amer. J. Physiol. 1992, 262: F494-498.

39.   Kambara, S., Yoshimura, M., Takahashi, H. & Ijichi, H.: Enhanced synthesis of renal dopamine ad impaired natriuresis in spontaneously hypertensive rats. Jpn. Heart J. 1987, 28:594 (abst.).

40.   Maemura, S., Niwa, M. & Ozaki, M.: Characteristic alterations in adrenal catecholamine content in SHR, SHRSP and WKY during development of hypertension and stroke. Jpn. Heart J. 1982, 23: 593-603.

41.   Racz, K., Kuchel, O., Buu, N.T. & Tenneson, S.: Peripheral dopamine synthesis and metabolism in spontaneously hypertensive rats. Circ. Res. 1985, 57: 889 - 897.

42.   Chen, C.J. & Lokhandwala, M.F.: An impairment of tubular DA-1 receptor function as the causative factor for diminished natriuresis to volume expansion in spontaneously hypertensive rats. Clin. Exp. Hypertnesion. 1992, 14(4): 615-628.

43.   DiBona, G.F.: Neural regulation of renal tubular sodium reabsorption and renin secretion: integrative aspects. Clin. & Exp. Hypertension. 1987, A9 (Suppl. 1): 151-165.

44.   Felder, R.A., Seikaly, M.G., Cody, P., Eisner, G.M. & Jose, P.A.: Attenuated renal response to dopaminergic drugs in spontaneously hypertensive rats. Hypertension. 1990, 15: 560-569

45.   Chen, C.J., Vyas, S.J., Eichberg, J. & Lokhandwala, M.F.: Diminished phospholipase-C activation by dopamine in spontaneously hypertensive rats. Hypertension. 1992, 19: 102-108.

46.   Kinoshita, S., Sidhu, A. & Felder, R.A.: Defective dopamine-1 receptor adenylate cyclase coupling in the proximal convoluted tubules from the spontaneously hypertensive rats. J. Clin. Invest. 1989, 84: 1849-1858.

47.   Mordachowicz, G.A., Sheikh, H.D., Jo, O.D., Nord, E.P., Lee, D.B. & Yanagawa, N: Increased Na/H antiport activity in the renal brush border membrane of SHR. Kidney Int. 1989, 36 (4): 576-581.

48.   Chen, C.J., Vyas, S.J., Eichberg, J., Beach, R.E. and Lokhandwala, M.F.: Abolished dopamine-1 receptor mediated inhibition of renal tubular Na^+,K^+-ATPase activity in spontaneously hypertensive rats. In: Genetic Hypertension. J. Sassard (ed). Colloque INSERM/John Libbey Eurotext Ltd, France; 218: 463-465, 1992.

49.   Felder, R.A., Kinoshita, S., Sidhu, A., Dhbu, K. & Kaskel, F.J.: A r enal dopamine receptor defect in two genetic models of hypertension. Amer. J. Hypertension. 1990, 3:96S - 99S.

A Molecular Approach to the Study of Renal Dopamine Receptors in Hypertension

Robin A. Felder*, Ikuyo Yamaguchi*,
Akira Horiuchi*, Pedro A. Jose[†] and
Robert M. Carey[§]

*Department of Pathology; [§]Department of Medicine, University of
Virginia Health Sciences Center, Charlottesville, VA 22908;
[†]Department of Pediatrics, Georgetown University Medical Center,
Washington, DC 20007, USA

ABSTRACT

An aberrant renal dopaminergic system may play a role in the pathogenesis of some forms of essential hypertension. Both human and animal models of hypertension have altered renal dopamine production and/or post-first messenger defects. The Dahl salt sensitive rat, which has a decreased ability to generate dopamine in the kidney, and the spontaneously hypertensive rat (SHR), which has no such limitation, have a defective coupling of a dopamine-D_1 receptor to the G protein/adenylyl cyclase complex. This coupling defect is: (1) receptor specific, (2) organ and nephron segment selective and of (3) genetic origin. A consequence of the defective renal proximal tubular dopamine receptor/adenylyl cyclase coupling in SHR is a decreased ability of D_1 agonists to inhibit renal luminal Na^+/H^+ exchange activity and a resistance to the natriuretic effect of dopamine and D_1 agonists. This resistance in SHR is due in part to a decreased cAMP production, although with maturation, a post cAMP defect is acquired. Whether the defect is in the primary or tertiary structure of the receptor remains to be demonstrated.

Dopamine regulates the excretion of sodium by hemodynamic actions as well as a direct inhibitory effects on tubular sodium transport (1-4). During hydropenia and volume loading ($\cong 10\%$ body weight), dopamine is not an important endogenous natriuretic factor (5). However, during moderate sodium chloride loading or volume expansion ($\approx 5\%$ body weight), dopamine becomes an important intrarenal natriuretic hormone (1, 2, 5, 6). Under these conditions, the natriuretic effect of dopamine is probably exerted mainly by inhibiting tubular sodium transport (1, 2, 6). In vitro studies have begun to elucidate the mechanism of action of dopamine on sodium transport systems. In 1976, Desiah and Ho reported that dopamine inhibits Na^+/K^+ATPase activity in mouse brain (7). This finding was confirmed by Aperia et al and by Takemoto et al in the proximal convoluted tubule and cortical collecting duct of the rat respectively (4, 8). In subsequent studies, Aperia and Bertorello reported that dopamine inhibits Na^+/K^+ATPase activity via a cAMP dependent mechanism following stimulation of a D_1 type of receptor

(9). Cyclic AMP, via protein kinase A, apparently inhibits Na^+/K^+ATPase activity by phosphorylating the α subunit of Na^+/K^+ATPase (10). In the thick ascending limb of Henle and probably the proximal tubule, this action is enhanced by the production of a protein phosphatase inhibitor (DARPP-32) which prevents the dephosphorylation of the sodium pump (11). In the proximal convoluted tubule dopamine, via a D_1 receptor, cAMP, and protein kinase A, also inhibits the luminal Na^+/H^+ exchanger (12, 13). In this nephron segment, dopamine via a D_1 type receptor also stimulates phospholipase C activity independent of its action on adenylyl cyclase (14-16). Protein kinase C, presumably produced in response to stimulation of phospholipase C by dopamine has also been shown to inhibit Na^+/K^+ ATPase activity (17). To date, studies have not determined how these actions of dopamine are regulated in a concerted manner through one or two different receptors with one or multiple signal transducing mechanisms.

Renal dopamine and hypertension

Dopamine can regulate blood pressure by actions in the central and peripheral nervous system (18) as well as target endocrine (e.g. adrenal glands) and transporting organs (e.g. kidney). Because some forms of hypertension are dependent or aggravated by sodium loading and because dopamine is an intrarenal natriuretic hormone, it has been postulated that an aberrant renal dopaminergic system may play a role in the pathogenesis of some forms of hypertension (2). Table 1 compares the relative concentration of renal dopamine and the natriuretic response to dopamine administration in human and some animal models of hypertension.

TABLE 1

Renal/Urine Dopamine Levels	Natriuretic Response to Dopamine/agonists	Animal Model	Human Counterpart
Normal/High (19)	Decreased (20,21)	SHR	Saito et al (22)
Low (19)	Decreased (23)	Dahl salt sensitive rat	?Clark et al (24)
Low (25)	Increased (26)	?Belgian SHR	Harvey et al (27) Kikuchi et al (28) Kuchel & Shigetomi (29) Yoshimura et al (30)

? = indirect evidence

In general, in human hypertensives whose renal dopamine levels are low and do not increase with sodium chloride loading, the natriuretic effect of exogenously administered dopamine is exaggerated (27-30). Black hypertensive subjects in particular have low urinary dopamine levels and do not increase in response to sodium loading (31). A group of human hypertensives in whom protein loading does not stimulate renal dopamine production may have an impaired natriuretic response to endogenous renal dopamine (24). There is a second group of patients with "sodium dependent" hypertension who have normal urinary dopamine levels (32, 33). The natriuretic effect of dopamine in these subjects has not been tested. Saito et al has reported that the urinary dopamine excretion of normotensive subjects with or without a family history of hypertension are similar but in those with a family history of hypertension, the positive correlation between urinary dopamine and sodium is lost (22). A third group of hypertensive patients who have elevated urinary dopamine levels are apparently resistant to the hypertensive effects of sodium loading (33).

Animal models of hypertension have also been reported to have "abnormal" urinary (or renal) dopamine levels (19). The natriuretic effect of dopamine is diminished in the Dahl salt sensitive rat which has decreased renal dopamine levels when compared to the Dahl salt resistant rat (23). The spontaneously hypertensive rat of the Okamoto/Aoki strain has been reported to have elevated renal dopamine levels (19, 30). With the exception of one preliminary report (26), these animals have a decreased natriuretic response to endogenous dopamine or exogenously administered dopamine or D_1 agonists (20, 21).

Renal Dopaminergic Defect in SHR

What mechanism(s) could be responsible for the attenuated natriuretic response to dopamine in some animal models of genetic hypertension? It is unlikely to be due to renal hemodynamic factors since the D_1 agonists increase renal blood flow to a similar extent in SHR and its normotensive controls, the Wistar-Kyoto rat (WKY). We, therefore, concentrated our efforts in determining the renal tubular mechanisms involved in this attenuated natriuretic response to dopamine. We reported that D_1 receptors (determined by radioligand binding with ^{125}I-SCH 23982) are most abundant in the renal cortex and are quantitatively and distributed similarly in WKY and SHR (20). More specifically, D_1 receptor density is similar in the proximal convoluted tubule and cortical collecting duct of 12-20 week old WKY and SHR (34, 35). However, the ability of dopamine and D_1 agonists to stimulate adenylyl cyclase activity in renal proximal tubules is decreased in the SHR (34, 36) in spite of a similar ability of guanyl nucleotides or forskolin to stimulate adenylyl cyclase activity in the proximal tubules of these rats (34).

Thus, the decreased ability of D_1 agonists to stimulate adenylyl cyclase in renal proximal tubules of SHR is not due to a defective enzyme per se or G protein but rather due to a defect in the coupling between a D_1 receptor and the G-protein/adenylyl cyclase complex. A defective coupling between a renal D_1 type receptor and phospholipase C has also been described in the SHR (21). Whether this defect is primary or secondary to the D_1/adenylyl cyclase defect remains to be determined.

The coupling defect is receptor specific since the ability of parathyroid hormone to stimulate adenylyl cyclase activity in proximal convoluted tubules is similar in WKY and SHR (34). It is also organ selective since D_1 agonists stimulate adenylyl cyclase activity in brain striatum to a similar extent in WKY and SHR (unpublished studies). It is also nephron segment selective since no differences in D_1 receptor density or affinity or adenylyl cyclase response to D_1 agonist stimulation in cortical collecting ducts are noted in WKY and SHR (35). This defect is probably of genetic origin since it is observed in the pre hypertensive state, i.e. young rats or rats fed a low salt diet (23, 34). For example, studies from our laboratory revealed that the D_1 receptor/adenylyl cyclase coupling defect in renal proximal convoluted tubules is present as early as 3 to 4 weeks of age before the onset of hypertension. In the WKY, the ability of D_1 agonists to stimulate adenylyl cyclase activity in proximal convoluted tubules increases with age (3-20 weeks); no such ontogenic response is seen in the SHR (34). We concluded from these studies that there is a maturational process in the coupling between the D_1 receptor and adenylyl cyclase in the proximal tubule of the WKY which does not occur in the SHR.

Other animal models of hypertension

We and others have also found a D_1 receptor/adenylyl cyclase coupling defect in the renal proximal convoluted tubule of Dahl salt sensitive rats (23, 37). However, these studies should be interpreted with caution since there are inherent problems with interstrain comparisons (38). Many of the physiologic and biochemical differences between hypertensive and normotensive strains have been explained by genetic drift and random fixation of alleles at loci that may not be involved in blood pressure regulation (39). Because fortuitously fixed characteristics in the SHR such as hyperactivity and hyper-reactivity to stress detract from the suitability of the SHR as a model for genetic hypertension, Hendley et al initiated a recombinant inbreeding program to create two new strains of SHR (40). One strain, the WK-HA, exhibits the hyperactive phenotype without the hypertension, and the other strain exhibited the hypertension without the accompanying hyperactivity, the WK-HT (40). We found the D_1 receptor/adenylyl cyclase coupling defect in the renal proximal convoluted tubule of the WK-HT but not in the WK-HA strain (41). Although classical cross-breeding experiments were not performed in these studies, these data support a genetic basis for a D_1 receptor/adenylyl cyclase coupling defect in renal proximal tubules in spontaneous hypertension.

Biochemical Studies of the Renal D_1 Receptor in Hypertension

Guanyl nucleotides regulate agonist interaction with antagonist labeled receptors in many adenylyl cyclase-coupled receptor systems (42). Presumably, guanyl nucleotides promote the dissociation of the receptor and the guanine nucleotide regulatory protein (G_s) resulting in a reduced affinity of the receptor for agonists. In proximal tubules from WKY, the ability of D_1 agonists to compete for specific ^{125}I-SCH-23982 (D_1 antagonist) binding sites is biphasic; the high affinity site has an inhibition constant of $1.8 \pm 0.8 \times 10^{-8}M$ while the low affinity site has an inhibition constant of $7.6 \pm 1.1 \times 10^{-5}M$. The addition of Gpp(NH)p (a non-hydrolyzable form of guanyl nucleotide) converts all to the binding to the low affinity site. N-ethyl maleimide, which alkylates sulfhydryl groups, also converts all the binding sites to the low affinity site; an effect that is prevented by prior treatment with a D_1 agonist. By contrast, only the low affinity site is detected in the SHR, the binding of which is unaffected by either Gpp(NH)p or N-ethyl maleimide (43).

We have also studied the solubilized D_1 receptor from rat renal proximal tubules. (34, 44). Photoaffinity labeling studies (using ^{125}I-MAB, a D_1 antagonist) revealed that the renal D_1 receptor has a molecular mass of 72-74 K dalton (34). In addition, two other minor bands, with Mr of 50 and 32 K are also present. In bovine parathyroid gland, ^{125}I-MAB is incorporated into polypeptide bands with Mr of 74, 62 and 51 K (45). Competition experiments (D_1 agonist vs ^{125}I-SCH-23982) using the solubilized receptor also reveals high and low affinity binding sites in the WKY but only a low affinity binding site is noted in the SHR. Similar to the studies using membrane bound receptors, guanyl nucleotides convert all of the binding sites to low affinity sites in the WKY; no such effect is noted in the SHR (34, 44). Therefore, the renal proximal tubular D_1 receptor from the SHR seems to be conformationally constrained into the low affinity state.

Sodium Transport Studies and the Renal D_1 Receptor in Hypertension

What role might an aberrant renal dopaminergic system play in the pathogenesis of some forms of hypertension? Since renal sodium handling is important in the initiation and/or maintenance of hypertension, we studied Na^+/H^+ exchange activity (a D_1 regulated transporter) in renal brush border membranes (43). As expected, the D_1 agonist, fenoldopam, or cAMP inhibits Na^+/H^+ exchange activity in renal brush border membrane vesicles in 12 week old WKY (12, 43). However, no such inhibitory effect is seen in the SHR. A decreased ability of dopamine to inhibit the antiporter in renal proximal tubules of SHR has also been reported (36). In other studies, we found that the ability of guanyl nucleotides (e.g. GTPγS) to inhibit the antiporter is not different between the SHR and WKY, supporting the notion of defect at the receptor site (46). The inability of cAMP to inhibit the exchanger in 12 week old SHR is surprising, and indicates a post-receptor defect, as well. However, since cAMP inhibits the antiporter to a similar extent in WKY and SHR at 3 weeks of age, we concluded that the resistance to the effect of D_1 agonists on sodium transport in the SHR is mainly due to decreased cAMP production; a post cAMP defect is acquired with maturation (43).

Molecular Biology of the Renal D_1 Receptors in Hypertension

Five different dopamine receptors have now been identified using molecular biologic techniques (2). Two of the subtypes (D_{1A} and D_{1B} also known as D_5) are each coupled to the stimulation of adenylyl cyclase and correspond to the classically described D_1 receptor. The D_2, D_3, and D_4 receptors are coupled to the inhibition of adenylyl cyclase and correspond to the classically described D_2 receptor. A D_1 dopamine receptor linked to stimulation of phospholipase C activity has not yet been cloned. All of the dopamine receptors cloned in brain are also expressed in tissues outside the central nervous system. The D_{1A}, D_{1B}, and D_3 receptor genes are expressed in specific nephron segments (47-49). The D_4 receptor gene is expressed in the heart (50). Limited studies using ribonuclease protection assays and sequencing of the 3rd cytoplasmic loop of the D_{1A}, D_{1B}, and $D_{2\text{-long}}$ receptors (amplified by PCR techniques with genomic DNA or mRNA from proximal tubules) have not yet detected any differences between WKY and SHR (48, 49). Thus, it remains to be seen whether there is a mutation in receptor segments not yet studied. Alternatively, a defect in the tertiary structure of a D_1 type receptor may be present in the SHR. Although previously activated deglycosylated receptors retain ligand binding activity (51), post-translational activation of receptors does require N-glycosylation. Glycosylation is a prerequisite for the acquisition process but after the receptor has acquired ligand binding activity, its N-linked oligosaccharide chains are no longer important for receptor activation. Such a mechanism may explain the results of our N-ethyl maleimide experiments if a defect in the primary structure of a D_1 type receptor is not uncovered with more extensive studies of the receptor. This may also explain the organ and nephron selectivity of the defect unless a defective D_1 receptor that is specifically expressed in the renal proximal tubule is discovered in spontaneous hypertension.

Conclusion

Hypertension is a multifactorial disease. However, in some types of hypertension, a coupling defect between the renal proximal tubular D_1 receptor and adenylyl cyclase may be responsible for the sodium retention noted in SHR and Dahl salt sensitive rats. Future studies will focus on defining the molecular mechanism of the receptor defect and its relation to sodium transport.

REFERENCES

1. Felder, R.A., Felder, C.C., Eisner, G.M., Jose, P.A. The dopamine receptor in adult and maturing kidney. Am J Physiol. 1989; 257: F315-F327.

2. Jose, P. A., Raymond, J.R, Bates, M.D., Aperia, A., Felder, R.A., Carey, R.M. The renal dopamine receptors. J Am Soc Nephrol. 1992; 2: 1265-1278.

3. Bello-Reuss, E., Higashi, Y., Kaneda, Y. Dopamine decreases fluid reabsorption in straight portions of rabbit proximal tubule. Am J Physiol. 1982; 242: F634-F640.

4. Aperia, A., Bertorello, A., Seri, I. Dopamine causes inhibition of Na^+-K^+-ATPase activity in rat proximal convoluted tubule segments. Am J Physiol. 1987;252: F39-F45.

5. Hansell, P., Fasching, A. The effect of dopamine receptor blockade on natriuresis is dependent on the degree of hypervolemia. Kidney Int. 1991; 39: 253-258.

6. Siragy, H. M., Felder, R.A., Howell, N. L.,Chevalier, R. L., Peach, M.J., Carey, R. M. Evidence that intrarenal dopamine acts as a paracrine substance at the renal tubule. Am J Physiol. 1989; 257: F469-F477.

7. Desaiah, D., Ho, I.K. Effect of biogenic amines and GABA on ATPase activities in mouse tissue. Eur J Pharmacol. 1976; 40: 255-261.

8. Takemoto, F., Satoh, T., Cohen, H. T., Katz, A. I. Localization of dopamine-1 receptors along the microdissected rat nephron. Pflugers Arch. 1991; 419: 243-248.

9. Bertorello, A., Aperia, A. Inhibition of proximal tubule Na^+-K^+-ATPase activity requires simultaneous activation of DA_1 and DA_2 receptors. Am J Physiol. 1990; 259: F924-F928.

10. Bertorello, A.M., Aperia, A., Walaas, S.I., Nairn, A.C., Greengard, P. Phosphorylation of the catalytic subunit of $Na+/K+ATPase$ inhibits the activity of the enzyme. Proc Natl Acad Sci USA. 1991; 88: 11359-11362.

11. Aperia, A., Fryckstedt, J., Svensson, L. , Hemmings, H. C. ,Jr., Nairn, A. C.,Greengard, P. Phosphorylated Mr 32,000 dopamine- and cAMP-regulated phosphoprotein inhibits Na^+,K^+-ATPase activity in renal tubule cells. Proc Natl Acad Sci USA. 1991; 88: 2798-2801.

12. Felder, C.C., Campbell, T. , Albrecht, F., Jose, P.A. Dopamine inhibits Na^+-H^+ exchanger activity in renal BBMV by stimulation of adenylate cyclase. Am J Physiol. 1990; 259: F297-F303.

13. Gesek, F.A., Schoolwerth, A.C. Hormonal interactions with the proximal Na^+-H^+ exchanger.

Am J Physiol. 1990; 258: F514-F521.

14. Felder, C.C ., Blecher, M., Jose, P.A. Dopamine-1 mediated stimulation of phospholipase C activity in rat renal cortical membranes. J Biol Chem. 1989; 264: 8739-8745.

15. Felder, C.C., Jose, P.A. Axelrod, J. The dopamine-1 agonist, SKF 82526, stimulates phospholipase-C activity independent of adenylate cyclase. J Pharmacol Exp Ther. 1989; 248: 171-175.

16. Vyas, S. J., Eichberg, J., Lokhandwala, M. F. Characterization of receptors involved in dopamine-induced activation of phospholipase-C in rat renal cortex. J Pharmacol Exp Ther. 1992; 260: 134-139.

17. Bertorello, A., Aperia, A. Na^+-K^+-ATPase is an effector protein for protein kinase C in renal proximal tubule cells. Am J Physiol. 1989; 256: F370-F373.

18. Sowers, J.R., Golub, M.S., Berger, M.E., Whitfield, L.A. Dopaminergic modulation of pressor and hormonal responses in essential hypertension. Hypertension. 1982; 4: 424-430.

19. Kuchel, O., Racz, K., Debinski, W., Falardeau, P., Buu, N.T. Contrasting dopaminergic patterns in two forms of genetic hypertension. Clin Exp Hypertens. 1987; A9: 87-1008.

20. Felder, R. A., Seikaly, M. G., Cody, P., Eisner, G.M., Jose, P.A. Attenuated renal response to dopaminergic drugs in spontaneously hypertensive rats. Hypertension, 1990; 15: 560-569.

21. Chen, C. J., Vyas, S. J. , Eichberg, J., Lokhandwala, M.F. Diminished phospholipase C activation by dopamine in spontaneously hypertensive rats. Hypertension. 1992; 19: 102-108

22. Saito, I., Takeshita, E., Saruta, T., Nagano, S., Sekihara, T. Urinary dopamine excretion in normotensive subjects with or without family history of hypertension. J Hypertens. 1986; 4: 57-60.

23. Nishi, A., Eklof, A-C., Bertorello, A., Aperia, A. Dopamine downregulation of proximal tubule Na^+, K^+-ATPase activity is lacking in Dahl salt sensitive rats. J Am Soc Nephrol. 1991; 2: 481

24. Clark, B.A., Rosa, R.M., Epstein, F.H., Young, J.B., Landsberg, L. Altered dopaminergic responses in hypertension. Hypertension. 1992; 19: 589-594.

25. Schoors, D.F., Dupont, A.G. Effect of carbidopa on the renal response to sodium loading in Wistar Kyoto and spontaneously hypertensive rats. Am. J. Hypertens. 1991; 4: 17A.

26. Schoors, D.F., Dupont, A.G. Increased renal response to fenoldopam in spontaneously hypertensive rats. Br J Pharmacol. 1989; 98: 747P.

27. Harvey, J.N., Casson, I.F., Clayden, A.D., Cope, G.F., Perkins, C.M., Lee, M. R. A paradoxical fall in urine dopamine output when patients with essential hypertension are given added dietary dalt. Clin Sci. 1984; 67: 83-88.

28. Kikuchi, K., Miyama, A., Nakao, T., Takigami, Y., Kondo, A., Mito, T., Ura, N., Tsuzuki, M., Iimura, O.. Hemodynamic and natriuretic response to intravenous infusion of dopamine in

patients with essential hypertension. Jpn Circ J. 1982; 46: 486-493.

29. Kuchel, O.,Shigetomi, S. Defective dopamine generation from dihydroxyphenylalanine in stable essential hypertensive patients. Hypertension. 1992;19: 634-638.

30. Yoshimura, M., Ikegaki, I. , Nishimura, M., Takahashi, H. Role of dopaminergic mechanisms in the kidney for the pathogenesis of hypertension. J Auton Pharmacol. 1990; 10: Suppl. 1: s67-s72.

31. Sowers, J.R., Zemel, M. B., Zemel, P., Beck, F.W.J., Walsh, MF., Zawada, E. T. Salt sensitivity in blacks. Salt intake and natriuretic substances. Hypertension. 1988; 12: 485-490.

32. Gordon, M.S., Steunkel, C A., Conlin, P.R., Hollenberg, N.K., Williams, G.H. .The role of dopamine in non-modulating hypertension. J Clin Endocrinol Metab.1989; 69: 426-432.

33. Gill, J.R., Jr., Gullner, H.G., Lake, C.R., Lakatua, D.J., Lan, G. Plasma and urinary catecholamines in salt-sensitive idiopathic hypertension. Hypertension. 1988; 11: 312-319.

34. Kinoshita, S., Sidhu, A., Felder, R. A. Defective dopamine-1 receptor adenylate cyclase coupling in the proximal convoluted tubule from the spontaneously hypertensive rat. J Clin Invest. 1989; 84: 1849-1856.

35. Ohbu, K., Felder, R.A. Nephron segment specificity of dopamine receptor/adenylyl cyclase defect in spontaneous hypertension. Am J Physiol. (in press).

36. Gesek, F.A., Schoolwerth, A.C. Hormone responses of proximal Na^+-H^+ exchanger in spontaneously hypertensive rats. Am J Physiol. 1991; 261: F526-F536.

37. Felder, R.A., Kinoshita, S., Sidhu, A. , Ohbu, K., Kaskel, F.J. A renal dopamine-1 receptor defect in two genetic models of hypertension. Am J Hypertens. 1990; 3: 96S-99S.

38. Rapp, J.P. Use and misuse of control strains for genetically hypertensive rats. Hypertension. 1987: 10: 127-131.

39. Kurtz, T. W., St. Lezin, E. M. Gene mapping in experimental hypertension. J Am Soc Nephrol. 1992; 3: 28-34.

40. Hendley, E.D., Ohlsson, W.G. Two new inbred strains derived from SHR: WKHA, hyperactive, and WKHT, hypertensive, rats. Am J Physiol. 1991; 262: H583-H589.

41. Ohbu, K., Felder, R.A. Renal dopamine-1 (DA-1) receptors from renal proximal convoluted tubules (PCT) of hypertensive normoactive rats. J Am Soc Nephrol. 1990;1:500.

42. Hess, E. J., Creese, I. Biochemical characterization of dopamine receptors. in Dopamine Receptors, Creese, I., Fraser, C. M., (editors) Alan R. Liss, Inc., New York, 1987, 1-27.

43. Horiuchi, A., Albrecht, F.E., Eisner, G.M., Jose, P.A., Felder, R.A. Renal dopamine receptors and pre- and post-cAMP mediated sodium transport defect in the spontaneously hypertensive rat. Am J Physiol. (in press).

44. Sidhu, A., Vachvanichsanong, P. , Jose, P.A., Felder, R. A. Persistent defective coupling of

dopamine- 1 receptors to G proteins after solubilization from kidney proximal tubules of hypertensive rats. J Clin Invest. 1992; 89: 789-793.

45.   Niznik, H.B., Fogel, E.L., Chen, C.J. , Congo, D. , Brown, E. M. , Seeman, P. Dopamine D1 receptors of the calf parathyroid gland: Identification and characterization. Mol Pharmacol. 1988; 34: 29-36.

46.   Albrecht, F.E., Felder, C.C., Eisner, G.M., Jose, P.A. Decreased dopamine (D_1) agonist inhibition of renal Na^+/H^+ exchange activity in spontaneous hypertension is due to a defect in the receptor and not to G protein. J. Am. Soc. Nephrol. 1992; 3: abstract.

47.   Yamaguchi, I., Jose, P.A., Mouradian, M.M., Canessa, L.M., Monsma, F.J. Jr., Sibley, D.R., Takeyasu, K., Felder, R.A. Expression of the dopamine D_{1A} receptor gene in the proximal tubule of the rat kidney. Am J Physiol. (in press).

48.   Jose, P. A., Monsma, F.J., Jr., Sibley, D.R., Mouradian, M.M., Felder, R.A. Significance of the D_{1A} and D_{1B} receptor mRNA in renal proximal tubules in Wistar Kyoto (WKY) and spontaneously hypertensive rat (SHR). Am J Hypertens. 1992; 5: 6A.

49.   Gao, D-Q., Monsma, F.J., Jr., Sibley, D.R., Canessa, L.M., Mouradian, M.M., Jose, P.A. Dopamine $D_{2\text{-long}}$ receptor gene expression in specific nephron segments demonstrated by reverse transcriptase (RT)/polymerase chain reaction (PCR). J Am Soc Nephrol . 1992; 3: abstract.

50.   O'Malley, K.L., Harmon, S., Tang, L., Han, S., Todd, R.D. The rat dopamine D4 receptor: sequence, gene structure, and demonstration of expression in the cardiovascular system. New Biol. 1992; 4: 137-146.

51.   Olson, T.S., Lane, M.D. A common mechanism for posttranslational activation of plasma membrane receptors? FASEB J. 1989; 3: 1618-1624.

Endogenous Digitalis-like Substance and Renal Dopaminergic System in Reduced Renal Mass Hypertensive Rat

Kazuaki Shimamoto, Hidehisa Nakagawa,
Motoya Nakagawa, Shigeyuki Saitoh,
Shin-ichiro Satoh and Osamu Iimura

Second Department of Internal Medicine, Sapporo Medical College,
S-1 W-16, Chuo-ku, Sapporo 060, Japan

Key words: Hypertension, Reduced renal mass rat,
DLS, DLF, Dopamine, Salt, Na-K ATPase

ABSTRACT

The pathophysiological significance of endogenous digitalis-like substance (DLS) and the renal dopaminergic system on blood pressure elevation was investigated in saline drinking reduced renal mass (RRM) rats. The hemi-nephrectomized (3/6 RRM), additional partially kidney resected (4/6RRM, 5/6 RRM), and sham operated (control) male Sprague-Dawley rats received 1% NaCl for 4 weeks.

Systolic blood pressure was elevated significantly during the 1st week in 5/6 RRM and continued to increase gradually until the 4th week, while no elevation in blood pressure was found in the other three groups. Urinary DLS increased immediately after the initiation of 1% saline drinking in all groups, except the control group, and returned to the basal level 2 weeks later in 3/6 and 4/6 RRM. Only in 5/6 RRM, did the urinary DLS remain augmented throughout 1 % NaCl drinking. A significant positive correlation was observed between urinary DLS and systolic blood pressure (r=0.28, p<0.05) in 5/6 RRM rats. The basal urinary dopamine (DA) excretion was significantly lower in the 3/6,4/6 and 5/6 RRM rats than in the control. After 1 % saline drinking, urinary DA increased in 3 RRM groups, while differences disappeared in the control and RRM rats. In 5/6 RRM rats, an increase in urinary DA continued throughout the experiment.

From these findings, it was suggested that in 5/6 RRM, DLS might have an important role in blood pressure elevation, and renal DA system may have a compensatory action to sodium retention and blood pressure increase.

INTRODUCTION

We have performed a series of experiments to investigate disturbances in sodium handling in essential hypertension, especially in low renin essential hypertension (1). Recently, we reported that decreases of urinary excretion of dopamine, kallikrein and prostaglandin E2, and augmented responses of urine volume, urinary sodium excretion, fractional excretion of sodium, urinary excretion of kallikrein and prostaglandin E2 to infused dopamine were recognized in essential hypertensives, and these decreases and augmentations were particularly obvious in the low renin group (1-3). Moreover, the suppression of this system was confirmed at the prehypertensive stage of essential hypertension (4). From these results, the possibility has been suggested that a reduction of renal dopaminergic activity exists, and this might be related to a disturbance of renal water-sodium handling in essential hypertension, especially in low renin essential hypertension.

It has been widely discussed whether chronic plasma volume expansion causes blood pressure elevation by increasing a "natriuretic hormone" involved in the regulation of renal sodium excretion (5). Plasma extracts of volume-expanded subjects inhibit microsomal Na-K ATPase, and therefore, this "natriuretic hormone" has been called a digitalis-like substance (DLS) (6). There is no doubt that DLS is observed in human plasma (7,8), and that plasma DLS is elevated in patients with essential hypertension (9). From these findings, the possibility exists that the genetic disturbance of renal sodium handling may induce volume expansion, and this expanded plasma volume stimulates DLS excretion, which results in natriuresis and a peripheral vascular resistance increment (10,11).

It is generally accepted that reduced renal mass (RRM) rats with high salt intake shows hypertension through volume expansion (12-13). In the present study, RRM hypertensive rats were employed as a sodium retention animal, and the pathophysiological role of DLS and renal dopaminergic system were investigated.

MATERIALS AND METHODS

Male Sprague-Dawley rats weighing 130-150 g were divided into the following 4 groups. 1/3 upper pole (4/6 RRM, n=16) or 1/3 both poles (5/6 RRM, n=13) of the left kidney was resected, and one week later, the right kidney was removed. One week after a sham operation, the right kidney was resected (3/6 RRM, n=12) or a second sham operation was repeated in control rats (control, n=13). Operations were performed under ether anesthesia.

After the second operation, rats were housed in metabolic cages and fed regular rat chow throughout the experiment. All rats were kept under constant temperature (20°C) with lights on and off every 12 hours. All rats were given tap water to drink for 1 week as a control interval before the experimental period. In the experimental period, all rats were given 1 % NaCl as drinking fluid until the end of the experiment. Urine was collected every 24 hours for 2 days at the end of the control period, and at the end of the 1st, 2nd, 3rd and 4th weeks after starting 1 % NaCl ingestion . Blood was taken from the abdominal aorta under ether anesthesia at the end of the experiment.

Urine volume (UV) and body weight were measured on the days of urine collection. Urinary sodium concentration was determined by the ion electrode method. Urinary immunoreactive DLS was measured by using a digoxin radioimmunoassay method previously reported from our laboratory (14). Briefly, urine was extracted with a Sep-Pak C-18 cartridge (Waters associates, Milford, MA) and eluted by ethanol. Extracted samples were incubated with digoxin antiserum provided from Mallinckrodt, Inc. (St. Louis, MO). The ^{125}-I digoxigenin was purchased from Dinabot Co. Ltd., Tokyo. Urinary free dopamine concentration(UDA) was determined by the HPLC-CDI method. Systolic blood pressure (SBP) was measured weekly by the tail-cuff method. The values of UV, urinary excretion of sodium (UNaV), UDA and urinary DLS excretion were expressed as the mean of 2 days urine collection. Serum creatinine level was measured by the Jaffe's method.

Statistical Analysis: Values were expressed as mean ± SEM. Statistical analyses between groups, and between weeks were performed by one-way analysis of variance (ANOVA). The null hypothesis was rejected when p value was less than 0.05.

RESULTS

UV and UNaV remarkably increased during the first week after 1 % saline drinking in all groups, except for UV in the control, which had a slight increase. In 3/6 and 4/6 RRM, both UV and UNaV decreased after the first week, while, on the other hand, in 5/6 RRM, UV and UNaV continued to increase until the 3rd week. UV and UNaV were higher in the order of 5/6, 4/6, 3/6 RRM and control throughout the experiment.

Only in 5/6 RRM did SBP increase significantly at the first week after 1 % NaCl drinking, and it continued to increase throughout the four weeks, but there was no significant change in SBP in the other 3 groups (Fig.1). Urinary DLS was slightly, but significantly, higher in 5/6 and 4/6 RRM at the end of the control period, during which all rats were given tap water to drink. After 1 % NaCl drinking, urinary DLS increased significantly in the 3/6, 4/6 and 5/6 RRM groups, but not in the control group. However, by the second week, urinary DLS had returned to the basal level in 3/6 and 4/6 RRM. In 5/6 RRM urinary DLS remained higher than the basal and the control group levels throughout the experiment . There was a significant positive correlation in 5/6 RRM between urinary DLS and SBP (r=0.28, p<0.05) and between urinary DLS and UNaV (r=0.66, p<0.01).

UDA was significantly lower in the 3/6, 4/6 or 5/6 RRM rats than in the control at the basal state before saline loading (Fig.2). After 1 % saline drinking, UDA was increased in 3/6, 4/6, or 5/6 RRM rats, and significant differences in each group disappeared at 1 week after saline drinking (data not shown). However, UDA returned to the basal level in 3/6 or 4/6 RRM rats at 2 and 3 weeks after 1 % saline drinking. In

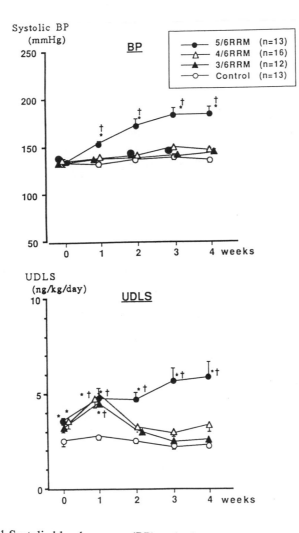

Fig.1 Systolic blood pressure (BP) and urinary endogenous digitalis-like
       substance excretion (UDLS) in control, 3/6, 4/6, and 5/6 RRM rats
       at control and at 1-4 weeks during the 1 % saline drinking.
       *; p<0.05 vs control   †; p<0.05 vs week O

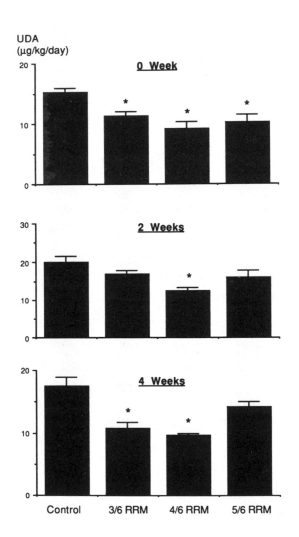

Fig.2 Urinary dopamine excretion (UDA) in control, 3/6, 4/6 and 5/6
     reduced renal mass (RRM) rats at basal state (0 week), 2 weeks
     and 4 weeks after 1 % saline drinking.
     *; $p < 0.05$ vs control

the 5/6 RRM hypertensive rats, UDA remained higher than in 3/6 and 4/6 RRM rats in the 3rd and 4th week after saline (Fig.2).

At the end of the experiment, the serum creatinine level was slightly, but significantly (p<0.05), higher in 5/6 RRM rats than in control rats, while no difference was found between RRM groups (0.47 ± 0.02, 0.57 ± 0.04, 0.61 ± 0.02 and 0.65 ± 0.04 mg/dl: control, 3/6, 4/6 and 5/6 RRM, respectively).

DISCUSSION

Although the pathophysiology of essential hypertension has been widely studied, the etiology of this disease is still unclear. Recently, it has been emphasized that essential hypertension might be linked to abnormal sodium handling. We reported that the renal depressor and natriuretic systems composed of dopaminergic, kallikrein-kinin and prostaglandin systems were suppressed in essential hypertensives , and the suppression of these systems may have an important pathophysiological significance in the etiology of hypertension through the retention of sodium and body fluid (1-3). In RRM hypertensive rats, UDA was suppressed only at the basal state. However, UDA increased temporally to the control levels after 1 % saline drinking in 3 RRM groups. In 5/6 RRM rats, the increased UDA continued throughout the experiment. These data suggested that renal DA system may contribute to the defense mechanism against the hypertension and the retention of sodium and body fluid in the 5/6 RRM hypertensive rats.

The natriuretic hormone, DLS, is considered to inhibit ouabain sensitive Na-K ATPase existing in both renal tubular and arteriolar smooth muscle, and the inhibition of this enzyme in the latter may lead to a rise in intracellular sodium and, consequently, calcium. Thus, DLS may increase vascular resistance and blood pressure. Several groups have demonstrated that plasma from hypertensive patients contains high levels of DLS which is assayed by either red cell or white cell cation flux (15,16), or by Na-K ATPase inhibition (11,17). 5/6 RRM rats have been known to be hypertensive in response to excess sodium intake. Huot et al. (18) reported a 19 % reduction of ouabain sensitive ^{86}Rb uptake at 1 week and a 40 % reduction at 5 weeks after subtotal nephrectomy in RRM hypertensive rats. Shima et al. (19) reported that plasma DLS measured by use of digoxin radioimmunoassay was higher in RRM hypertensive rats than in control rats. The authors previously reported that a transient increase of DLS in 4/6 and 3/6 RRM rats failed to elevate the blood pressure (14). In this study, increased DLS was found in established 5/6 RRM hypertension. Although urinary DLS excretion increased significantly in 3/6 and 4/6 RRM rats during the first week, they did not show hypertension. On the other hand, in 5/6 RRM rats urinary DLS continued to increase during the 1 % NaCl drinking. Furthermore, in 5/6 RRM rats, SBP was raised significantly at the first week and continued to be elevated throughout the experiment. This observation suggests that high DLS levels might maintain high blood pressure in 5/6 RRM hypertensive rats. A significant positive correlation between DLS and SBP seems to support this conclusion as well. Consequently, there was a significant positive correlation between DLS and SBP and between DLS and UNaV. These results indicate that urinary DLS seems to be related to both the elevation of blood pressure and the augmentation of sodium excretion in 5/6 RRM rats.

From these data, it was concluded in RRM hypertensive rats that renal dopaminergic system may compensate the blood pressure increase and sodium retention, and that DLS may play an important role in the excretion of sodium, and the continuous augmentation of DLS may be neccesary to induce blood pressure elevation in 5/6 RRM rats.

ACKNOWLEDGMENT

This work was supported by the Ministry of Health and Welfare "Adrenal Hormone" Research Committee, and also by the Kanae Foundation of Research for New Medicine, 1991.

REFERENCES

1. Iimura O, Pathophysiological significance of sympathetic function in essential hypertension. Clin Exp Hypertens 1989; A11(Suppl): 103-115

2. Iimura O, Kikuchi K, Yamaji I, The pathophysiological role of renal dopaminergic activity in patients with essential hypertension. Jpn Circ J 1987; 51:1232-1240

3. Iimura O, Shimamoto K, Ura N, The pathophysiological role of renal dopamine, kallikrein-kinin and prostaglandin systems in essential hypertension. Agents and Actions 1987; 22:247-256

4. Iimura O, Shimamoto K, Ura N, Dopaminergic activity and water-sodium handling in the kidneys of essential hypertensive subjects: Is renal dopaminergic activity suppressed at the prehypertensive stage ? J Cardiovasc Pharmacol 1990; 16(Suppl 7):S56-S58

5. de WardenerHE, MacGregor GA, Dahl's hypothesis that a saluretic substance may be responsible for a sustained rise in arterial pressure; its possible role in essential hypertension. Kidney Int 1980; 18:109

6. Gonick HC, Krammer HJ, Paul W, Lu E, Circulating inhibitor of sodium-potassium activated adenosine triphosphatase after expansion of extracellular fluid volume in rats. Clin Sci Mol Med 1977; 53:329-334

7. Kramer HJ, Pennig J, Digoxin-like immunoreacting substance(s) in the serum of patients with chronic uremia. Nephron 1985; 40:297-302

8. Graves SW, Valdes R, Jr, Brown BA, Endogenous digoxin-immunoreactive substance in human pregnancies. J Clin Endocrinol Metab 1984; 58: 748-751.

9. Saitoh S, Shimamoto K, Nakagawa M, Yamaguchi Y, Matsuda K, Kuroda S, Ura N, Iimura O, The pathophysiological role of digitalis-like substance in essential hypertension. J Hypertens 1988; 6 (suppl 4): S360-S362.

10. de Wardener HE, Millet J, Holland S, MacGregor G, Alaghband-Zadeh J, The endogenous cytochemically assayable Na-K ATPase inhibitor and its relation to hypertension. Klin Wochenschr 1987; 65 (suppl VIII): 4-7.

11. Hamlyn JM,Ringel R, Schaeffer J, Levinson PD, Hamilton BP, Kowarski AA, Blaustein MP, A circulating inhibitor of Na-K ATPase associated with essential hypertension. Nature 1982; 300: 650-652.

12. Pitcock J, Brown P, Brooks B, Clapp W, Brosius M, Muirhead E, Renomedullary deficiency in partial nephrectomy-salt hypertension. Hypertension 1980; 2: 281-290.

13. Ylitalo P, Gross F, Hemodynamic changes during the development of sodium induced hypertension in subtotally nephrectomized rats. Acta Physiol Scand 1979; 106: 447-455.

14. Nakagawa M, Shimamoto K, Matsuda K, Saitoh S, Nakagawa H, Ura N and Iimura O, The transient increase of urinary digitalis-like substance excreted during excess sodium intake in reduced renal mass rats. Am J Hypertens 1990; 3: 873-875.

15. Edmondson RPS, Thomas RD, Hilton PJ, Patrick J, Jones NP, Abnormal leucocyte composition and sodium transport in essential hypertension. Lancet 1975; 1: 1003-1005.

16. Meyer P, Garay RP, Genetic markers in essential hypertension. Clin Exp Hypertension 1981; 3:4-8.

17. MacGregor GA, Teuton S, Alaghband-Zadeh J, Markandu N, Roulston JE, de Wardener HE, Evidence for a raised concentration of a circulating sodium transport inhibitor in essential hypertension. Br Med J 1981; 283: 1355-1357.

18. Huot SJ, Pamnani MB, Clough DL, The role of sodium intake, the Na-K pump and a ouabain-like humoral agent in the genesis of reduced renal mass hypertension. Am J Nephrol 1983; 3: 92-99.

19. Shima H, Masuyama Y, The increased activity of the sympathetic nervous system in pathogenesis of reduced renal mass-salt hypertension and its augmenting mechanism by humoral factor. J. Wakayama Med. Soc., 1988; 39 : 47-69.

Presence of Dopaminergic DA$_2$ Binding Sites in Pheochromocytoma

R. Lanzillotti*, C. Pupilli*, L. Ianni*, G. Fiorelli*,
R.M. Carey[+] and M. Mannelli*

*Department of Clinical Physiopathology, Endocrinology Unit,
University of Florence, viale Pieraccini 6, 50134 Florence, Italy
[+]University of Virginia, School of Medicine, Charlottesville,
Virginia, USA

ABSTRACT

To verify whether dopamine DA2 receptors are present in human pathological chromaffin cells, receptor binding study was performed in 2 unilateral adrenal pheochromocytomas using ^{3}H spiroperidol. Bovine adrenal medulla was used as control. Scatchard analysis of binding data obtained in bovine adrenal medulla demonstrated the presence of two different binding sites, one with high affinity (R1, Kd = 1.4 ± 0.4 x 10^{-10} M) and low capacity (6.2 ± 1.2 fmol/mg protein) and one with low affinity (R2, Kd = 1.6 ± 0.4 x 10^{-8} M) and high capacity (223 ± 47 fmol/mg protein). Similarly to bovine adrenal medulla, two binding sites were present in both pheochromocytomas, exhibiting different Kd and binding capacities.
Our data demonstrate the presence of dopamine DA2 receptor binding sites in pheochromocytoma tissue. The activation of these receptors might represent the mechanism through which DA2 receptor antagonists cause hypertensive crises in pheochomocytoma patients.

INTRODUCTION

Dopaminergic DA2 receptors have been demonstrated in chromaffin tissue of several species by receptor binding studies (1, 2). In vitro studies on isolated cat, bovine and rabbit adrenal glands have also demonstrated that DA2 receptor agonists were able to decrease catecholamine secretion induced by nicotine or splanchnic nerve stimulation (3-5). This inhibitory effect was reverted by DA2 receptor antagonists (3-5) and seemed to be mediated by a reduction in calcium uptake (6).

In an in vivo study carried out in normal male subjects, we demonstrated that during high simpathetic stimulation induced by physical exercise, the administration of domperidone, a DA2 receptor antagonist, significantly increased the amount of epinephrine secreted by the human adrenal medulla, suggesting a modulatory role for adrenal DA2 receptors in these experimental conditions (7).

Whether such a modulatory role is present also in pathological human chromaffin tissue is not known, although it has been reported that the administration of antidopaminergic agents, such as metoclopramide and sulpiride, in patients affected by pheochromocytoma can induce a secretory burst which in turn cause a hypertensive crisis (8, 9).

As a first step to investigate the mechanism through which antidopaminergic agents causes hypertensive crises in pheochromocytoma patients, we performed receptor binding studies on two pheochromocytomas. Bovine adrenal medulla was used as control.

MATERIALS AND METHODS

Pheochromocytoma tissues were obtained at surgery from 2 female patients (20 and 33 years old) affected by unilateral adrenal pheochromocytoma. Bovine adrenal medulla were obtained at the local slaughterhouse, put in ice-cold TRIS-HCl buffer (pH 7.4) and quickly tranferred to the laboratory were the adrenal medulla was carefully dissected out of the gland. Tissues were homogenized in ice-cold 50mM TRIS-HCl buffer (pH 7.4), containing 0.1 mM phenylmethyl-sulphonyl fluoride, 0.25 mM $CaCl_2$, 0.32 M sucrose, with a teflon-glass homogenizer and centrifuged at 300 g for 10 min. The pellet was discarded and the supernatant was centrifuged at 800 g for 20 min. Again, the pellet was discarded and supernatant was centrifuged at 100000 g for 60 min in a Beckman ultracentrifuge. The pellet was washed with 50 mM TRIS-HCl buffer (pH 7.4), containing 0.1 mM phenylmethyl-sulphonyl fluoride and 0.25 mM $CACl_2$ and centrifuged at 100000 g for 60 min. The final pellet was resuspended in the same buffer, divided in fractions and stored at -80 °C. The protein content of membrane samples was determined by a spectrophotometric method according to Bradford (10), using BSA as a standard. At the moment of the assay, membrane preparations (0.2 mg protein/ml) were resuspended in 50 mM TRIS-HCl buffer (pH 7.4) containing 120 mM NaCl, 5mM HCl, 1mM MgCl$_2$, 2mM CaCl$_2$, 10 uM pargiline, 0.1 % ascorbic acid and 5% BSA and preincubated at 22 °C for 30 min with 0.5 uM ketanserine, 1uM labetalol and 0.1uM phenoxybenzamine to block serotoninergic and adrenergic receptors. 200 ul of membrane samples in triplicate were than incubated at 22 °C for 60 min with increasing amounts (0.2-0.8 nM) of ^{3}H-spiroperidol (Amersham, Buckingamshire, U.K.; specific activity 118 Ci/mMol) in tubes without the unlabeled compound and with a fixed concentration (0.6 nM) of 3H-spiroperidol in tubes containing increasing concentrations (0.3-500 nM) of the unlabeled compound (saturation/displacement curve). The binding reaction was terminated by addition of cold TRIS-HCl buffer and samples were filtered through Whatman fiber glass filters GF/C (Whatman, Clifton, NJ). Filters were than washed twice with 5 ml cold buffer and radioactivity was counted in a Beckman liquid scintillation counter. Specific binding of ^{3}H-spiroperidol was calculated as the amount displaced by 500 nM spiroperidol. At 22 °C the non specific binding was around 50% of the total.

Experiments were carried out on two different pools of bovine adrenal medulla and repeated 4 times for each pool. Pheochromocytoma tissues were analyzed as single specimen. Scatchard analysis of binding data was performed using the computer program LIGAND.

RESULTS

Preliminary experiments were carried out to determine the best experimental conditions for 3H-spiroperidol binding to bovine adrenal membranes. Binding resulted time and temperature dependent. Although the maximal specific binding to 4 different membrane preparations was observed at 37 °C, binding at 22 °C resultend significantly more costant. Therefore, our study was carried out at this temperature. The effect of protein concentration on ^{3}H-spiroperidol binding was studied between 0.05 and 1.0 mg/ml and resulted linear in this range. Therefore, all subsequent assays were carried out using a protein concentration of 0.2 mg/ml. As graphically represented in Fig. 1 panel A, scatchard analysis of the results obtained in the bovine adrenal medulla using LIGAND showed that a model for 2 binding sites fitted the data significantly better than a model for a single binding site. As reported in table 1, these two classes of binding sites showed different Kd (R1=$1.4 \pm 0.4 \times 10^{-10}$ M and R2= $1.6 \pm 0.4 \times 10^{-8}$ M respectively) and different binding capacities (R1 = 6.2 ± 1.2 fmol/mg protein and R2 = 223 ± 47 fmol/mg protein, respectively).

Also in pheochromocytoma membrane preparations scatchard analysis showed the presence of two different binding sites (Fig 1, panel B). The result of scatchard analysis for each pheochromocytoma is reported in table 1.

TABLE 1

Scatchard Analisysis of Binding Data in Bovine Adrenal medulla (mean of 8 experiments) and in 2 Pheochromocytomas.

| | SITE 1 | | SITE 2 | |
	Kd $\times 10^{-10}$ M	Bmax fmol/mg prot	Kd $\times 10^{-8}$ M	Bmax fmol/mg prot
Bovine adrenal medulla	1.4 ± 0.4	6.2 ± 1.2	1.6 ± 0.4	223 ± 47
Pheochromocytoma patient 1	4.3	230	17	55000
patient 2	1.5	33	4.2	4304

Values are Mean ± SE.

In both pheochromocytoma the R1 binding site showed a Kd quite similar to that one found in bovine adrenal medulla while the Kd of R2 showed a higher variability.

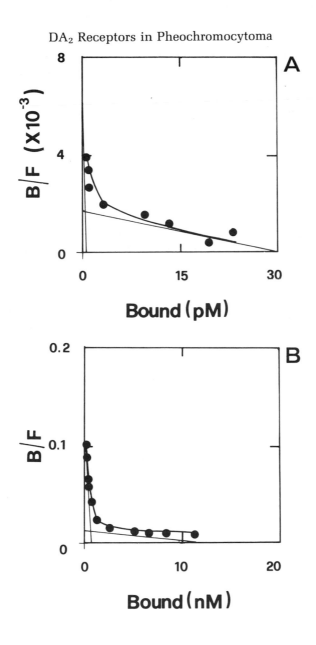

FIG. 1 Graphic representation of scatchard analysis of receptor binding data in bovine adrenal medulla (panel A) and in one pheochromocytoma (panel B). In both tissues, the curve was biphasic, indicating receptor heterogeneity.

At variance with the bovine adrenal medulla, the binding capacities of the 2 different tumors were highly variable.

DISCUSSION

Our data confirm the presence of specific spiroperidol (DA2) binding sites in bovine adrenal medulla and demonstrate that also human pheochromocytoma tissue posseses these binding sites.

The binding data from the two type of chromaffin tissues were analyzed using the computer program LIGAND for one- and two-class binding site model. The fitting of a two-site binding model to the data provided the best extimates (in the least square sense) demonstrating the presence of two binding sites, one with high affinity (Kd 10^{-10} M) and low capacity (R1) and one with lower affinity (Kd 10-8 M) and higher capacity (R2). These results are at variance with those of previous studies that found only one tipe of DA2 binding sites in bovine adrenal medulla (1, 2). This difference can be explained by differences in the experimental conditions such as the use of unlabeled spiroperidol to displace the radiolabeled tracer, the preincubation of membrane preparations with ketanserin and phenoxybenzamine, and the use of a saturation/displacement curve. Nevertheless, it is worth mentioning that, when our data are fitted for a one site binding model , the Kd results almost identical to that one previously reported (Kd= 0.09 nM).

From our data it is not possible to conclude whether the two sites represent two different affinity states of one receptor or two distinct receptors. Further studies will be necessary to address this point.

Similarly to bovine adrenal medulla, each pheochromocytoma tissue showed the presence of specific binding sites for spiroperidol, confirming the results obtained by our group using autoradiography (11). However, in the present study, the use of the saturation/displacement curve technique allowed us to reveal the presence of two different binding sites (R1, R2) with different affinities and capacities, in close agreement with the data obtained in the bovine adrenal medulla.

The mechanism through which antidopaminergic agents induce catecholamine secretion by pheochromocytoma cells is unknown. Theoretically, antidopaminergic agents might induce catecholamine secretion acting directly on DA2 receptors located on tumoral cells or on DA2 receptors located on noradrenergic nerve terminals repleted of circulating catecholamines. The demonstration of DA2 receptor binding sites on tumoral cells does not permit to exclude any of the above mentioned hypotheses.

Although not univocally (6,12,13), data from the literature seem to indicate that activation of DA2 receptors inhibits catecholamine release from normal chromaffin tissue by limiting intracellular calcium disposal. In vitro study are necessary to establish whether DA2 receptors regulate catecholamine release from pheochromocytoma cells through the same mechanism.

REFERENCES

1 Lyon, R.A., Titeler, M., Bigornia, L., Schneider, A.S. D2 dopamine receptors on bovine chromaffin cell membranes: Identification and characterization by (3H)N-methylspiperone binding. J Neurochem. 1987; 48: 631-635.

2 Quik, M., Bergeron, L., Mount, H., Philie, J. Dopamine D2 receptor binding in adrenal medulla: Characterization using 3H spiperone. Biochem Pharmacol. 1987; 36:3707-3713.

3 Collet, A.R., Story, D.F. Is catecholamine release from the rabbit adrenal gland subject to regulation through dopamine receptors or beta-adrenoceptors? Clin Exp Pharmacol Physiol. 1982; 9:436.

4 Artalejo, A.R., Garcia, A.G., Montiel, C., Sanchez-Garcia, P. A dopaminergic receptor modulates catecholamine release from the cat adrenal gland. J Physiol. 1985; 362: 359-368.

5 Gonzales, M.C., Artalejo, A.R., Montiel, C., Hervas, P.P., Garcia, A.G. Characterization of a dopaminergic receptor that modulates adrenomedullary catecholamine release. J Neurochem. 1986; 47: 382-388.

6 Bigornia, L., Suozzo, M., Ryan, K.A., Napp, D., Schneider, A.S. Dopamine receptors on adrenal chromaffin cells modulate calcium uptake and catecholamine release.J Neurochem. 1988; 51: 999-1006.

7 Mannelli, M., Pupilli, C., Fabbri, G., Musante, R., DeFeo, M.L., Franchi, F., Giusti, G. Endogenous dopamine (DA) and DA2 receptors: a mechanism limiting excessive sympathetic-adrenal discharge in humans. J Clin Endocrinol Metab. 1988; 66: 626-631.

8 Plouin, P.F., Menard, J., Corvol, P. Hypertensive crisis in patient with pheochromocytoma given metoclopramide. Lancet. 1976; 2: 1357-1358.

9 Marafelia, P., Perrot, L., Berthezene, F. Valeur semeiologique du test ou sulpiride et au glucagon dans le depistage du pheochromocytome. Rev Franc Endocrinol Clin. 1986; 27: 197-200.

10 Bradford, M.M. A rapid and sensitive method for qauntitation of microgam quantities of protein, utilizing the principle of protein-dye binding. Cancer. 1977;40:2257-2263.

11 Mannelli, M., Pupilli, C., Lanzillotti, R., Ianni, L., Amenta, F., Ricci, A., Serio, M. Dopamine modulation of pathological human chromaffin tissue. Am J Hypertens. 1990; 3: 22S-24S.

12 Huettl, P., Gerhardt, G.A., Browning, M.D., Masserano, J.M. Effects of dopamine receptor agonists and antagonists on catecholamine release in bovine chromaffin cells. J Pharmacol Exp Ther. 1991; 257: 567-574.

13 Sontag, J.M., Sanderson, P., Klepper, M., Aunis, D., Takeda, K., Bader, M.F. Modulation of secretion by dopamine involves decrease in calcium and nicotinic currents in bovine chromaffin cells. 1990; 427: 495-517.

Effects of Ibopamine on Cardiac Angiotensin Converting Enzyme (ACE) Activity in Different Experimental Models of Chronic Heart Failure

Dirk J. van Veldhuisen*, Wiek H. van Gilst[†],
Hendrik Buikema[†], Egbert Scholtens[†],
Pieter A. de Graeff[†], Bart J.G.L. de Smet[†],
Armand R.J. Girbes[‡], K.I. Lie*
and Harry Wesseling[†]

*Dept of Cardiology/Thoraxcenter; [†]Dept of Clinical Pharmacology;
[‡]Division of Intensive Care, Dept of Surgery, University Hospital,
Oostersingel 59, 9713 EZ Groningen, The Netherlands

ABSTRACT

The aim of this study was to investigate cardiac angiotensin converting enzyme (ACE) activity and plasma neurohumoral activation and the influence of ibopamine in different models of experimentally induced chronic heart failure (CHF). Accordingly, we studied 60 rats with myocardial infarction (MI) (n=20), aortic banding/stenosis (AS) (n=20) or no operation (normals) (n=20). Six weeks after surgery rats were randomly assigned to control treatment or ibopamine (10 mg/day) for 3 weeks.

At the end of the study, rats with MI and AS had significantly higher levels of plasma norepinephrine (PNE) than normal rats, but plasma epinephrine, aldosterone, renin and plasma ACE activity were equal in the 3 groups. Cardiac ACE-activity (non-infarcted left ventricle) was increased in rats with MI (12.1 ± 1.9 U/l/min), compared to normals (4.2 ± 0.2 U/l/min) and rats with AS (4.1 ± 0.3 U/l/min). Ibopamine treatment lowered PNE levels in both MI and AS, but not in normals. Other plasma neurohumoral parameters were also unaffected by the drug. Cardiac ACE-activity in MI rats was signficantly reduced by ibopamine (9.6 U/l/min; p< 0.05), but was unchanged in the other groups.

In conclusion, these 2 models of experimental CHF reflect different neurohumoral abnormalities. Ibopamine exerts neurohumoral modulating properties, both in plasma (PNE levels) and in cardiac tissue (ACE-activity).

INTRODUCTION

A variety of experimental and clinical models have shown that in addition to hemodynamic changes, neurohumoral activation is an important component in the sequence of increased wall stress, ventricular hypertrophy and dilatation, and subsequent remodeling and chronic heart failure (CHF) (1). Drugs that inhibit this vascular and/or tissue neuroendocrine activation may therefore be beneficial in the prevention or early treatment of CHF.

Ibopamine is an orally active, aselective dopamine agonist, with both hemodynamic and neurohumoral effects (2). Clinically, the drug mainly causes vasodilation and mild diuresis (3). In addition, ibopamine lowers plasma norepinephrine (PNE) concentrations, which may be secondary to its hemodynamic effect, but which also be caused by a direct (presumably DA-2) receptor mediated effect (2,4-6). The influence of ibopamine on the renin-angiotensin system is less clear. DA-2 receptor stimulation may cause inhibition of aldosterone secretion in the presence of sodium depletion (7,8), and a lowering effect on plasma renin has also been reported (9), although this was not confirmed by others (8). The purpose of the present study was to examine the influence of ibopamine on plasma and cardiac neuroendocrine activation in different models of experimental CHF.

METHODS

Sixty normotensive male Wistar rats (230-250 g), with myocardial infarction (MI; n=20), aortic stenosis/banding (AS; n=20) or no operation (normals; n=20) were studied. Six weeks after surgery, rats were randomized to ibopamine (10 mg/kg/day), or standard treatment for 3 weeks after which they were sacrificed. Ibopamine was dissolved in water and was given by gavage twice daily; the control group received the same amount of only water by gavage as well.

Operation techniques. Surgery was performed while rats were anaesthetized with 1-1.5% fluothane, intubated and ventilated mechanically. MI was induced by coronary ligation as described by Pfeffer et al (10). In our laboratory, this technique causes cardiac hypertrophy and pulmonary congestion (11) and a significant decrease in contractile response (12), indicating CHF. AS was made by the method of Linz et al (13), whereby a ligature is tightened around the aorta and a 23-gauge needle, just between the left and right renal artery. After the needle is removed, the aorta is constricted with a diameter of ± 0.65 mm. With this procedure, left ventricular hypertrophy occurs (13), and subsequent left ventricular dysfunction, as was shown by a significant decrease in contractile response (12).

Plasma neurohumoral measurements. PNE (with HPLC), plasma aldosterone and plasma renin activity (with radioimmunoassay) and plasma ACE-activity (with fluorometry) were all determined as previously described (14), at the end of the 9 week study (ie. 6 weeks following surgery, and 3 weeks with ibopamine/control treatment).

Cardiac ACE-activity determination. After the right ventricular free wall, the atria and the valves were cut off, the remaining cardiac tissue (left ventricle) was cut into 2 transverse pieces, of which the caudal one was used. This part mainly contained the non-infarcted apex, to minimize possible confounding effects of scar tisssue. The method we used for determination of tissue ACE-activity was the one described by Hirsch et al (15). In short, the tissue is rinsed, homogenized and diluted using different buffers. A substrate is then added, which is converted by ACE into His-Leu. Using fluorometry, the amount of His-Leu which is tagged by phtaldialdehyde, then relects the ACE-activity in the specimen.

Statistical analysis. Comparisons were made with unpaired Student's t tests and MANOVA was used in case of repeated measurements. Values are mean ± SEM and a p value < 0.05 was considered significant.

RESULTS

Of the 60 rats who were included, 11 died. The remaining 49 rats (23 controls, 26 ibopamine) finished the study and were analyzed (17 normals (8/9), 15 MI (8/7) and 17 AS rats (7/10).

Plasma neurohormones (Figure 1). PNE levels were higher in rats with MI (251 ± 19 pg/ml) and rats with AS (245 ± 26 pg/ml) compared to normal rats (203 ± 21 pg/ml) (both MI and AS vs. normals p< 0.05), but plasma aldosterone, plasma renin and plasma ACE-activity were neither increased in

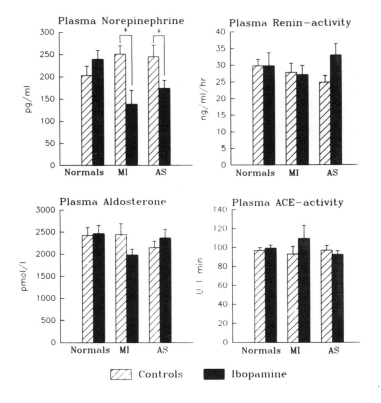

Figure 1: Plasma neurohumoral parameters. * p< 0.05

MI nor in AS rats. Treatment with ibopamine significantly reduced PNE levels in rats with MI (to 138 pg/ml) and rats with AS (174 ± 18 pg/ml), but had no signficant effects on PNE levels in normal rats. Other plasma neurohumoral parameters were also unaffected by ibopamine.

Cardiac ACE-activity (Figure 2). In rats with MI, cardiac ACE activity was signficantly increased (12.1 ± 1.9 U/l/min), but not in rats with AS (4.1 ± 0.3 U/l/min), compared to normal rats (4.2 ± 0.2 U/l/min). Ibopamine significantly reduced cardiac ACE-activity in rats with MI (9.6 U/l/min), but did not affect rats with AS or normal rats.

DISCUSSION

In this study we have investigated 2 different animal models of cardiac dysfunction/CHF. In both the MI and in the AS model, there was a decrease in contractile reserve (12) and PNE levels were elevated. In contrast, cardiac ACE-activity was increased only in the MI model. Ibopamine lowered PNE levels and cardiac ACE-activity, but only when these parameters were elevated.

Cardiac ACE-activity in our AS model was not increased, in contrast to previous reports, in which an increase in cardiac ACE-activity was observed in rats with aortic banding and pressure overload hypertrophy (16). Although the elevation of PNE levels and the reduction of contractile reserve (12) were similar in the AS and MI models, hemodynamically the 2 were different as both heart rate and blood pressure were higher in AS (12). CHF resulting from

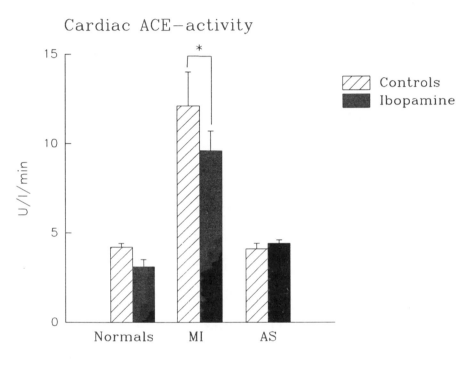

Figure 2: Cardiac ACE activity. * p< 0.05

pressure-overload may need a longer period to develop, and symptoms are different and sometimes less manifest than in CHF caused by myocardial infarction. Long-term pressure overload, as observed in hypertension and in this experimental AS model, induces left ventricular hypertrophy, which initially causes primarily diastolic dysfunction. CHF resulting from MI, however directly causes systolic dysfunction. Indeed, it is not clear which trigger induces an increase in ACE-activity in CHF, and whether this is more related to systolic or diastolic dysfunction. Furthermore, it would be interesting to evaluate the influence of ibopamine in an AS model with elevated cardiac ACE-activity.

The increase in cardiac ACE-activity in the MI model indicates local activation of the renin-angiotensinin system, despite the fact that plasma parameters of this system are normal. The latter finding is in accordance with clinical studies (17), in which plasma renin is usually normal in untreated CHF. When ACE-activity increases, angiotensin II concentrations will likely increase. Since angiotensin II induces cardiac hypertrophy (18), this increase in cardiac ACE-activity may be an important factor in the process of remodeling after MI. Indeed, the favorable effect of ACE-inhibitors on this process may well be attributed to their inhibiting effects on angiotensin II formation (19). Since ibopamine lowered the elevated ACE-activity in rats with MI and caused no long-term changes in heart rate and blood pressure (12), this suggests a direct modulating influence, either due to a local inhibitory effect on the renin-angiotensin system or to the decrease in PNE levels. Catecholamines also have a growth stimulating effect on the myocardium (20) and the combination of a

reduction in both PNE levels and cardiac ACE-activity may suggest a favorable

role for ibopamine in preventiing ventricular remodeling following myocardial

infarction.

REFERENCES

1.   Francis GS, McDonald M. Left ventricular hypertrophy: an initial
        response to myocardial injury. Am J Cardiol 1992; 69: 3G-9G

2.   Henwood JM, Todd PA. Ibopamine. A preliminary review of its pharma-
        codynamic and pharmacokinetic properties and therapeutic efficacy.
        Drugs 1988; 36: 11-31

3.   Rousseau MF, Raigoso J, Van Eyll C, Van Mechelen H, Musso NR,
        Lotti G, Pouleur H. Effects of epinine administration on left ventricular
        systolic performance, coronary hemodynamics, and circulating catechola-
        mines in patients with heart failure. J Cardiovasc Pharmacol 1992; 19:
        155-162

4.   Rajfer SI, Rossen JD, Douglas FL, Goldberg LI, Karrison T. Effects of
        long-term therapy with oral ibopamine on resting hemodynamics and
        exercise capacity in patients with heart failure: relationship to the
        generation of N-methyldopamine and to plasma norepinephrine levels.
        Circulation 1986; 73: 740-748

5.   Van Veldhuisen DJ, Crijns HJ, Girbes ARJ, Tobé TJM, Wiesfeld ACP,
        Lie KI. Electrophysiologic profile of ibopamine in patients with congesti-
        ve heart failure and ventricular tachycardia and relation to its effects on
        hemodynamics and plasma catecholamines. Am J Cardiol 1991; 68: 1194-
        1202

6.   Girbes ARJ, Van Veldhuisen DJ, Grevink RG, Smit AJ, Reitsma WD.
        Effects of ibopamine on exercise-induced increase in norepinephrine in
        normal men. J Cardiovasc Pharmacol 1992; 19: 371-374

7.   Carey RM, Thorner MO, Ortt EM. Effects of meteclopramide and bromocriptine on the renin-angiotensin-aldosterone system in normal man. J Clin Invest 1979; 63: 727-735

8.   Missale C, Metra M, Sigala S, Memo M, Dei Cas L, Spano PF. Inhibition of aldosterone secretion by dopamine, ibopamine, and dihydroergotoxine in patients with congestive heart failure. J Cardiovasc Pharmacol 1989; 14(suppl 8): S72-S76

9.   Nakano T, Morimoto Y, Kakuta Y, Konishi T, Kodera T, Kanamuru M, Takezawa H. Acute effects of ibopamine hydrochloride on hemodynamics, plasma catecholamine levels, renin activity, aldosterone, metabolism and blood gas in patients with severe congestive heart failure. ArzneimittelForschung 1986; 36: 1829-1834

10.   Pfeffer MA, Pfeffer JM, Fishbein MC, Fletcher PJ, Spadaro J, Kloner RA, Braunwald E. Myocardial infarct size and ventricular function in rats. Circ Res 1979; 44: 503-512

11.   Van Wijngaarden J, Monnink SHJ, Bartels H, Van Gilst WH, De Graeff PA, De Langen CDJ, Wesseling H. Captopril modifies the response of infarcted rat hearts to isoprenaline stimulation. J Cardiovasc Pharmacol 1992; 19: 741-747

12.   Van Veldhuisen DJ, Van Gilst WH, De Graeff PA, De Smet BJGL, Scholtens E, Buikema H, Girbes ARJ, Wesseling H, Lie KI. Different models of chronic heart failure in rats, and the influence of oral ibopamine (abstract). Eur Heart J 1992; 13(abstract suppl): in press

13.   Linz W, Schölkens BA, Ganten D. Converting enzyme inhibition specifically prevents the development and induces regression of cardiac hypertrophy in rats. Clin Exp Hypert 1989; A11: 1325-1350

14.   De Graeff PA, Kingma JH, Dunselman PHJM, Wesseling H, Lie KI. Acute hemodynamic and hormonal effects of ramipril in chronic congestive heart failure. Am J Cardiol 1987; 59(suppl D): 164D-170D

15.   Hirsch AT, Talsness CE, Scunkert H, Paul M, Dzau VJ. Tissue-specific activation of cardiac angiotensin converting enzyme in experimental heart failure. Circ Res 1991; 69: 475-482

16.   Lorell BH, Schunkert H, Grice WN, Tang SS, Abstein CS, Dzau VJ. Alteration in cardiac angiotensin converting enzyme activity in pressure overload (abstract). Circulation 1989; 80(suppl II): II-297

17.   Francis GS, Benedict C, Johnstone DE, Kirlin PC, Nicklas J, Liang CS, Kubo SH, Rudin-Toretsky E, Yusuf S, for the SOLVD Investigators. Comparison of neuroendocrine activation in patients with left ventricular dysfunction with and without congestive heart failure (SOLVD). Circulation 1990; 82: 1724-1729

18.   Naftilan AJ, Pratt RJ, Eldridge CS, Lin HL, Dzau VJ. Angiotensin II induces c-fos expression in smooth muscle via transcriptional control. Hypertension 1989; 13: 706-711

19.   Hirsch AT, Pinto YM, Schunkert H, Dzau VJ. Potential role of the tissue renin-angiotensin system in the pathophysiology of congestive heart failure. Am J Cardiol 1990; 66: 22D-32D

20.   Tarazi RC, Sen S, Saragoca M, Khairallah P. The multifactorial role of catecholamines in hypertensive cardiac hypertrophy. Eur Heart J 1982; 3(suppl A): 103-110

Further Studies on Gludopa in Man: The Effect of the Monoamine Oxidase Inhibitor Selegiline

S. Freestone, T.C. Li Kam Wa and M.R. Lee

Department of Clinical Pharmacology, The Royal Infirmary,
Edinburgh EH3 9YW, UK

ABSTRACT

The effect of the monoamine oxidase (MAO)-B inhibitor, selegiline, on the renal actions of the renal dopamine prodrug τ-L-glutamyl-L-dopa (gludopa) was studied in nine healthy men. Gludopa 15 μg kg^{-1} min^{-1} was infused intravenously for 3h after pretreatment with selegiline 20 mg or placebo. Gludopa infusion caused a 460-fold increase in urine dopamine excretion from 1.9 $\pm$ 1.2 to 875 $\pm$ 151 nmol min^{-1}. This was associated with an increase in urinary sodium excretion from 214 $\pm$ 66 to 485 $\pm$ 203 μmol min^{-1} (P < 0.01). Selegiline enhanced the increase in dopamine excretion and reduced the increment in 3,4-dihydroxyphenylacetic acid (DOPAC) excretion, the urinary dopamine/DOPAC ratio increasing significantly from 2.35 $\pm$ 0.51 to 2.96 $\pm$ 0.36 (P < 0.01). Selegiline did not change the natriuresis or the reduction in plasma renin activity (PRA) due to gludopa. Selegiline alone did not change urine sodium excretion or PRA. Inhibition of MAO-B reduces the conversion of dopamine to DOPAC in the kidney in man.

INTRODUCTION

τ-L-glutamyl-L-dopa (gludopa) is a renal dopamine prodrug sequentially converted by τ-glutamyl-transferase and L-amino acid decarboxylase to dopamine in the proximal renal tubule. As these enzymes have high relative activities in renal tissue the conversion is relatively specific for the kidney. The dopamine so formed acts on DA$_1$ and DA$_2$ receptors to induce natriuresis and renal vasodilation and to reduce PRA (1,2).

Dopamine is metabolised by several different routes:

(i) conjugation to form the sulphate or glucuronide conjugates

(ii) by MAO to DOPAC and

(iii) by catechol-O-methyltransferase (COMT) to 3-methoxytyramine and then by MAO to homovanillic acid.

In studies with selective MAO inhibitors using rat kidney slices it was concluded that both MAO-A and MAO-B are important in the metabolism of newly formed dopamine (3). Subsequently the same workers found that MAO-A and MAO-B activities were similar in the medulla of human kidneys and MAO-B activity was greater than that of MAO-A in the renal cortex. We have therefore investigated the effect of a selective MAO-B inhibitor, selegiline, on the renal metabolism and effects of gludopa. The hypothesis under test was that selegiline would inhibit the conversion of dopamine (generated from gludopa) to DOPAC and increase the effects of gludopa infusion.

METHODS

Nine healthy men aged $26.8 \pm$ (SD) 7.3 years and weighing 74.9 ± 8.8 kg were studied on 3 occasions. They were screened by physical examination and had normal haematology and plasma biochemistry results. They attended at 08.30h after an overnight fast, having abstained from caffeine containing drinks from 22.00h on the previous evening. They received 300 ml water with either selegiline 20 mg (on two occasions) or placebo tablets in random order. Thirty minutes later (time 0) bladder emptying occurred and subsequently eight accurately timed urine collections of about 45 minutes duration were made. 300 ml of water was taken by mouth after each bladder emptying. Subjects remained semi-recumbent except when passing urine. Blood pressure and heart rate were measured in duplicate by a Dinamap semi-automated recorder at 15 minute intervals. Venous blood was collected at 45 minute intervals via an indwelling cannula sited in the left antecubital fossa.

After two baseline urine collections (0-1.5h), gludopa 15 μg kg^{-1} min^{-1} in 0.9% sodium chloride [150 mmol l^{-1}; (saline)] or saline alone was infused at 0.5 ml min^{-1} intravenously in the opposite arm for 3 hours (1.5-4.5h) and after termination of the infusion two further urine collections were made (4.5-6h). The three combinations studied were selegiline 20 mg orally + gludopa infusion; placebo + gludopa infusion and selegiline 20 mg orally + saline infusion.

Sample Collection and Analysis

Blood samples for measurement of PRA were collected into pre-cooled tubes containing sodium EDTA and kept on ice before centrifugation at 4°C. Plasma was separated and stored at -40°C until analysis. PRA was measured by radioimmunoassay of angiotensin I generated under standard conditions (4). The intra-and inter-assay coefficients of variation were 4% and 6% respectively.

Urinary sodium concentrations were measured by an ion-selective electrode (Radiometer KNA1 Analyser). Urine samples for dopamine and DOPAC assay were acidified with 5M hydrochloric acid to prevent oxidation. Dopamine was extracted from urine onto alumina and eluted with 0.2M acetic acid by the method of Anton and Sayre (5). It was measured by high performance liquid chromatography (hplc) and electrochemical detection with epinine as internal standard, as previously described (1). Intra- and inter-assay coefficients of variation were < 4% and the lower limit of detection was 5 ng ml^{-1}. The extraction procedure for DOPAC was similar to that for dopamine except that elution occurred with 0.2M perchloric acid and dihydroxybenzylamine was used as internal standard.

Results were analysed by repeated measures analysis of variance and paired t test or Wilcoxon rank sum tests.

RESULTS

Administration of gludopa resulted in a 460-fold increase in urine dopamine excretion from a baseline value of 1.9 ± 1.2 nmol min^{-1} to 874.7 ± 151.3 nmol min^{-1} during the last 45 minutes of infusion (P < 0.001). Similarly DOPAC excretion increased from 3.0 ± 1.2 to 396.0 ± 107.7 nmol min^{-1} over the same time period (Table 1). Associated with this increase in urine dopamine, urinary sodium excretion rose from 213.8 $\pm$ 66.4 to a peak value 485.2 $\pm$ 203.1 μmol min^{-1} (P<0.01, Figure 1). PRA fell from 1.2 $\pm$ 0.6 ngAI ml^{-1} h^{-1} at baseline to 0.7 $\pm$ 0.4 ngAI ml^{-1} h^{-1} at the end of gludopa infusion (P<0.01). Blood pressure did not change significantly during gludopa infusion, being 119.4 $\pm$ 7.4/ 71.3 $\pm$ 9.0 mm Hg at baseline and 116.6 $\pm$ 8.1/ 68.6 $\pm$ 7.5 mm Hg during the last 45 minutes of infusion.

TABLE 1

Mean (SD) urinary dopamine and DOPAC excretion (nmol min^{-1}) and dopamine/DOPAC ratio (n=9).

Urine collection	1	2	3	4	5	6	7	8
Gludopa alone								
Dopamine	2.0	1.9	312.5	672.6	793.1	874.7	544.7	258.5
	(1.0)	(1.2)	(29.1)	(87.4)	(97.1)	(151.3)	(82.2)	(117.2)
DOPAC	3.5	3.0	114.6	269.7	355.4	396.0	270.0	137.6
	(1.8)	(1.2)	(34.9)	(86.9)	(106.5)	(107.7)	(71.8)	(61.2)
Dopamine/DOPAC ratio	0.65	0.68	2.92	2.65	2.38	2.31	2.10	2.02
	(0.34)	(0.41)	(0.73)	(0.65)	(0.62)	(0.48)	(0.40)	(0.59)
Gludopa + Selegiline								
Dopamine	1.9	2.2	329.1	680.1	878.9	958.7	594.3	254.4
	(0.8)	(1.0)	(55.4)	(116.7)	(150.7)	(136.5)	(103.2)	(57.7)
DOPAC	3.6	3.6	94.9	236.1	297.0	311.0	228.8	94.2
	(2.0)	(1.8)	(23.5)	(39.0)	(40.6)	(59.7)	(47.9)	(22.1)
Dopamine/DOPAC ratio	0.64	0.67	3.54	2.93	2.99	3.15	2.63	2.77
	(0.33)	(0.38)	(0.41)	(0.58)	(0.51)	(0.61)	(0.30)	(0.67)

After pretreatment with selegiline 20 mg, urine dopamine excretion increased from 2.2 $\pm$ 1.0 to a peak of 958.7 $\pm$ 136.5 nmol min^{-1} during the last 45 minutes

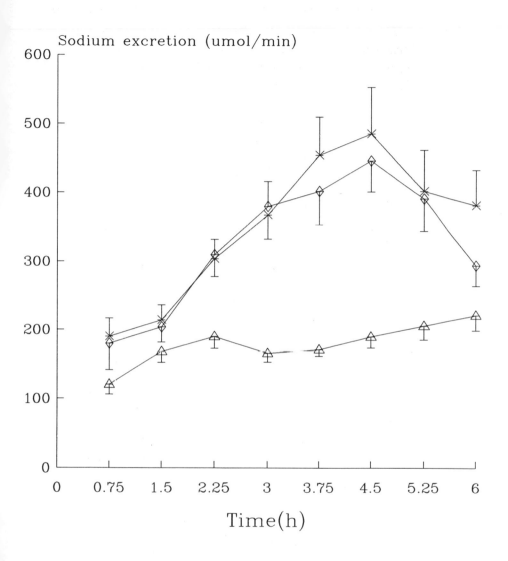

FIG. 1   Urine sodium excretion (mean and sem) in 9 normal subjects.
x = placebo + gludopa, ♦ = selegiline + gludopa, ▲ = selegiline + saline

S. Freestone et al.

of gludopa infusion. DOPAC excretion rate rose over this period from 3.6 ± 1.8 to 311.0 ± 59.7 nmol min^{-1}. Cumulative dopamine excretion in urine over the period of gludopa infusion and 1.5h afterwards (1.5-6h) was increased by 7% from 155.5 to 166.3 μmol (P < 0.05) after pretreatment with selegiline. Similarly cumulative (1.5-6h) urinary DOPAC excretion was reduced by 18% from 69.5 to 56.8 μmol (P < 0.05) in the presence of selegiline. The mean dopamine/DOPAC ratio in urine collected over this time was significantly increased by selegiline pretreatment from 2.35 ± 0.51 to 2.96 ± 0.36, an increase of 26% (P < 0.01). Despite the increase in urinary dopamine the natriuretic effect of gludopa was not enhanced by selegiline pretreatment, urine sodium excretion increasing from 203.9 ± 66.5 μmol min^{-1} at baseline to a peak of 445.7 ± 134.3 μmol min^{-1} at the end of gludopa infusion. The fall in PRA with gludopa remained significant (P < 0.05) but was also not enhanced by selegiline (0.9 ± 0.8 ngAI ml^{-1} h^{-1} at baseline vs 0.6 ± 0.3 ngAI ml^{-1} h^{-1} at 4.5h, P < 0.05).

Saline infusion after oral selegiline 20 mg did not cause any significant change in urine dopamine or DOPAC excretion and did not increase sodium excretion rate or reduce PRA.

DISCUSSION

Intravenous infusion of gludopa caused the expected increase in urine dopamine excretion, natriuresis and reduction in PRA, as seen in previous studies in our department (1,2,6). Fernandes and Soares-da-Silva (3) showed that newly formed dopamine can be deaminated by both MAO-A and MAO-B. Pretreatment with the selective MAO-B inhibitor, selegiline, resulted in an 18% reduction in urine DOPAC excretion and a small but statistically significant increase in dopamine excretion. Consequently after selegiline pretreatment the urine dopamine/DOPAC ratio was higher at all times during and after infusion of gludopa. However despite the increase in urine dopamine excretion, neither the natriuretic effect of gludopa nor the reduction in PRA was enhanced by selegiline. This is probably due to the high concentrations of dopamine produced in response to gludopa in this dose (a 460-fold increase from baseline levels) and consequently saturation of renal dopamine receptors in the presence or absence of selegiline. In addition the increase in urinary dopamine excretion after selegiline pretreatment was only modest; this is possibly due to metabolism along alternative pathways, for example by COMT or by conjugation.

In conclusion selective inhibition of MAO-B with selegiline does reduce the conversion of dopamine (produced from gludopa) to DOPAC by the kidney in vivo in man. The effect of selective MAO-A inhibition on this process in man has still to be determined.

REFERENCES

1. MacDonald TM, Jeffrey RF, Freestone S, Lee MR. (+)-sulpiride antagonises the renal effects of τ-L-glutamyl-L-dopa in man. Br J Clin Pharmacol 1988, **25**, 203-212.

2. Worth DP, Harvey JN, Brown J, Worral A, Lee MR. Domperidone treatment in man inhibits the fall in plasma renin activity induced by intravenous τ-L-glutamyl-L-dopa. Br J Clin Pharmacol 1986, **21**, 497-502.

3. Fernandes MH, Soares-da-Silva P. Effects of MAO-A and MAO-B selective inhibitors Ro 19-1049 and Ro 19-6327 on the deamination of newly formed dopamine in the rat kidney. J Pharmacol Exp Ther 1990, **255**, 1309-1313.

4. Haber E, Koerner T, Page LB, Kliman B, Purnode A. Application of a radioimmunoassay for angiotensin I to the physiological measurement of plasma renin activity in normal human subjects. J Clin Endocrinol Metab 1969, **29**, 1349-1355.

5. Anton AH, Sayre DF. The distribution of dopamine and dopa in various animals and a method for their determination in diverse biological material. J Pharmacol Exp Ther 1964, **145**, 326-336.

6. Jeffrey RF, MacDonald TM, Marwick K, Lee MR. The effect of carbidopa and indomethacin on the renal response to τ-L-glutamyl-L-dopa in normal man. Br J Clin Pharmacol 1988, **25**, 195-201.

Dopamine Prodrugs in Cardiovascular and Renal Disease

C. Casagrande

Zambon Research S.p.A., Bresso, Milan, Italy

ABSTRACT

Prodrugs of dopamine carrying various protecting moieties have been designed for improved absorption and protection from first-pass metabolism, and also for selective delivery to target organs. Ibopamine and docarpamine are examples of prodrugs acting orally on peripheral dopamine receptors, as opposed to levodopa, acting both centrally and peripherally. Ibopamine, a prodrug of epinine, owes its beneficial effects in congestive heart failure to both DA_1 and DA_2 receptor stimulation. Gludopa and Sim 2055, as examples of prodrugs endowed with a good degree of renal selectivity, are useful tools in the investigation of the pathophysiological and therapeutic relevance of dopaminergic mechanisms in the kidney.

INTRODUCTION

The observation by Goldberg and associates (1) of the natriuretic and renal

vasodilator effects of an intravenous infusion of dopamine (DA) in congestive

heart failure (CHF) patients was the starting point of research leading to the

therapeutic application of DA infusion but also to the identification of specific

receptors mediating the effects of DA in the cardiovascular and renal system, and

to extensive investigation of the physiological role of endogenous DA in normal

and in pathological conditions. These developments have been reviewed (2).

Essentially, two main subtypes of peripheral receptors, currently classified as

DA_1 and DA_2, are present in the kidney, in the adrenal cortex, in the arterial bed

and in sympathetic nerves (probably including a class of dopaminergic nerves)

and ganglia, and exert control of cardiovascular and renal homeostasis directly,

by inhibition of Na^+ reabsorption and aldosterone secretion and by vasodilation,

particularly in the renal and mesenteric bed, and indirectly by reducing sympa-

© 1993 Pergamon Press Ltd.
Printed in Great Britain.

thetic tone. The classification of peripheral DA receptors is being expanded by the recognition of new subtypes, taking advantage of increasing knowledge of the structure of the receptors and the mechanisms of signal transduction, in parallel with the discovery of new subtypes of DA receptors in the central nervous system (CNS) (3).

In the aim of widening the applications of DA, various groups investigated new agonist of DA receptors (2). Other groups, including our own, endeavoured to improve the pharmacokinetic properties of DA by converting it into prodrugs designed to overcome the lack of absorption and short duration of action, and additionally to achieve selective delivery to target organs, in order to improve efficacy and avoid side effects (4). The prodrug approach has been proposed as a practicable way of improving the properties of many classes of drugs. Scrutiny of the literature shows however that therapeutically useful achievements have been more limited than predicted. Catecholamines are highly polar endogenous substances eliciting effects in many organs, and also undergoing a rapid metabolic inactivation in the same organs, in relationship to their role of neuronal and hormonal mediators. Thus, improvements in terms of absorption, duration of action, and specific site delivery could be expected from the physical, chemical and metabolic modifications attainable by the synthesis of prodrugs. However, only two adrenergic prodrugs have shown clinical usefulness, and both by topical application only: dipivefrine, the dipivaloyl ester of dl-epinephrine instilled in the eye for the treatment of glaucoma, and bitolterol, the di-p-toluyl ester of N-t-butyl-dl-norepinephrine, administered by inhalation as a long lasting bronchodilator (4).

In general, applications of prodrugs have been successful in solving pharmaceutical problems such as poor taste, irritation at the site of application, lack of solubility or stability, or modulation of the rate of dissolution, and also in improving the diffusion through a local barrier in topical use. The rate of success rapidly decreased when problems of systemic bioavailability, high first pass metabolism, or short duration of action had to be faced, and even more when selective delivery was required. These are indeed the problems to be solved in the case of DA-prodrugs; a survey of the present status of their development shall be preceded by a brief analysis of the pharmacokinetic and metabolic determinants of prodrug actions. Compartmental, physiological, and hybrid models are available to this purpose (5, 6): a suitable model is represented in Fig. 1, where a central compartment, comprehensive of the pharmacologically neutral compartments, is linked to a target compartment (T) and to a compartment expressing side effects (S). Each compartment is characterized by its own rate parameters of prodrug (P) to drug (D), conversion (V_{max} and K_m) and volume of distribution (V), which may differ for P and D, as shown in the case of the central compartment. Transfer of prodrug and drug to and from the T and S compartments, as well as elimination, have individual kinetic characteristic, expressed by clearance terms (Cl_{in}, Cl_{out}, and Cl_{el}). A variety of simulations (5, 6), including the use of physiological parameters, such as the fractions of cardiac output (CO) perfusing the T and S compartments, brings into evidence the main determinants. Systemic bioavailability is enhanced by fast absorption and low first pass metabolism (included in the term Cl_{el}^{P}), preferentially followed by fast conversion of P into D in the central and/or the target compartment, with relatively slow elimination of the drug (low Cl_{el}^{D}). A smaller volume of distribution of the prodrug (V^{P}) with respect to the drug (V^{D}) favours the transfer of the first to the active compartments. Fast diffusion of the prodrug, which is also dependent on the rate of perfusion of the T compartment, has moderate effects and lacks selectivity, since

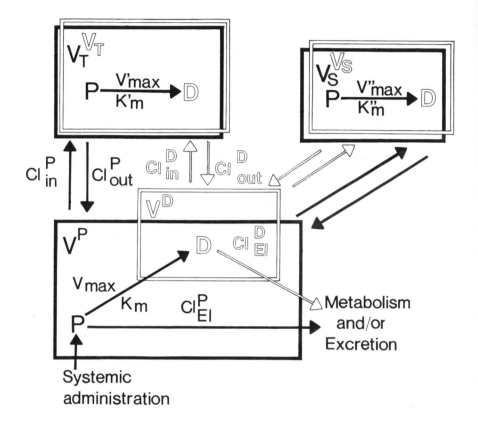

FIG. 1 - Pharmacokinetic model of distribution and activation of systemic prodrugs. See text for explanation.

diffusion to other compartments shall also be fast, as well as back-diffusion; a markedly more favourable role is played by its active uptake in the T compartment. A major determinant of selectivity is the retention of the drug in the target organ, while the binding or retention of the prodrug may also contribute, as far as it does not hinder the conversion of P into D.

Formulae of DA prodrugs discussed in the present paper are shown in Fig. 2. A comprehensive review of their properties is available (4).

IBOPAMINE

Ibopamine (IBO), the 3,4-diisobutyryl ester of epinine (N-methyldopamine) was selected from a series of prodrugs of DA and N-substituted DA analogues in which esterification of the catechol system was used to increase lipophilicity and decrease first-pass conjugation. The selection criteria referred to the ability of the prodrugs to reproduce, on oral administration, all the effects of an i.v. infusion of DA (4). Hemodynamic investigations in anesthetized dogs showed that IBO increased renal blood flow, without any change in other parameters at doses as low as 0.8-2 mg/kg, comparably to i.v. DA at 1-2.5 μg/kg min. The effect on renal circulation and urine excretion were increased dose proportionally up to 24 mg/kg. Left ventricular dP/dt and CO were increased in dose related way starting from 6 mg/kg, with a simultaneous but less marked increase in mean arterial pressure. Systemic vascular resistance (SVR) was unchanged at 8-12 mg/kg and reduced at 24 mg/kg; these effect matched those of i.v. DA at 5-20 μg/kg min, a noticeable difference being that IBO slightly reduced heart rate, whereas DA increased it. The onset of action was rapid and the effects lasted 1-3 hours, depending on the dose and the parameters considered. Dose-dependent diuretic and natriuretic effects of oral IBO in rats (2.5 - 100 mg/kg) were similar to those of i.p. administered DA (0.5-4 mg/kg). These effects were suppressed by d-sulpiride.

In various experimental models IBO was virtually devoid of CNS effects on peripheral administration, differing from levodopa, used for comparison as a DA precursor able to cross the blood-brain barrier, but it was markedly active when administered intracerebrally. Tissue distribution studies showed that IBO, although lipophilic, did not penetrate the CNS because of fast conversion to polar epinine by ubiquitous esterases in peripheral tissues.

Clinical hemodynamic investigations of orally administered IBO confirmed the laboratory results showing that vasodilation and increase of CO induced by 100-200 mg of the drug in CHF patients were comparable to those of 2-4 μg/kg min of DA, and lasted 5-6 hours. While only modest diuretic and natriuretic effects were observed with doses of 50-100 mg of IBO in healthy volunteers, marked and clinically significant effects were shown daily in a 7-day treatment of CHF patients with 50 mg bid, along with an increase in creatinine clearance. An important contribution to the beneficial effects of IBO derived from the its ability to counteract the neurohumoral activation typical of CHF, by inducing a sustained reduction of plasma norepinephrine (NE) and aldosterone; plasma renin activity (PRA) also tended to decrease. Thus, both DA_1 and DA_2 receptors appear to mediate the clinical action of IBO; contribution of presynaptic α_2-adrenoceptors cannot be excluded. Several controlled trials proved the ability of IBO, at a dose of 100 mg tid, to improve clinical conditions and functional capacity of CHF patients in chronic treatment, as well as its substantial safety, particularly in the lack of arrhythmogenic risk. The usefulness shown in these trials is supported by the results of Phase IV studies in Italy and the Netherlands, where the drug is commercially available (4, 7).

In addition to the application in CHF, preliminary studies indicate a therapeutic potential of IBO in chronic progressive renal failure and in peripheral arterial disease. Alleori et al. (8) showed in the latter condition an increase in leg blood flow velocity which was antagonized by sulpiride, along with an increase of walking ability. In a study in patients of chronic renal failure, change in slope of the serum creatinine concentration curve was observed in two sequential 6-month periods, respectively without and with IBO treatment, indicating that the progression of the renal impairment was significantly delayed (9).

DOCARPAMINE

Docarpamine (DOC) is a prodrug of DA protected by esterification of the catechol function, similarly to IBO, and additionally by a metabolically reversible acylation of the amino group with N-acetylmethionine, probably affording a degree of protection from MAO during absorption. Since DOC can be activated by esterases and amidases or peptidases in various tissues, it cannot be expected to show organ selectivity. In hemodynamic studies in dogs it showed dopaminergic, β-adrenergic and α-adrenergic effects in sequence, similar to DA and IBO, by increasing doses ranging from 3.7 to 33.5 mg/kg i.d.   Emetic effects were weaker than those of levodopa (10). Pharmacokinetic studies showed that the prodrug is deesterified during absorption, yielding N-acetyl-L-methionyldopamine, which is peripherally circulated along with free DA with a half-life of 0.6 hours (11). When DOC was directly injected into the renal artery, specific renal activation was not observed, confirming the view that the renal effects of low doses of DOC depend on circulating DA (12).

DOC is reported to be in active development for the chronic treatment of CHF in high doses (750 mg tid or qid). Reports are currently limited to acute and short term treatment (4). In an invasive hemodynamic study (12) doses of 750-1500 mg moderately but significantly increased cardiac index (CI) (13%) and decreased SVR (15%) for 2 hours leaving other parameters unchanged. Urine volume and glomerular filtration rate were increased in the first hour while renal plasma flow (RPF) was increased up to three hours. Similar renal effects were observed in severe CHF after a single dose of 1200 mg (13). Controlled trials of chronic treatment are now awaited to confirm the therapeutic potential of this prodrugs.

LEVODOPA

Levodopa, as used in Parkinson disease, is an example of a prodrug explaiting specific transport systems for absorption and transfer into its target organ; selectivity is improved when peripheral metabolism (V_{max}) is depressed by coadministration of peripheral inhibitors of dopadecarboxylase. CNS retention of DA, owing to neuronal mechanisms of active uptake and storage and to a small rate of outflow, is probably contributing as well.

Some investigations of levodopa were conducted in CHF patients, limited as expected by side effect such as diskinesia, nausea and vomiting (4). In two studies by Rajfer et al. (14, 15) levodopa showed significant hemodynamic effects, which were maintained in a chronic treatment of 3 months, or longer. Typically, 1.5 g of levodopa acutely increased CI by 30% and decreased SVR by 25% . Symptomatic improvement was also reported in the chronic treatment. The plasma levels of NE were not decreased, neither acutely nor chronically; it was therefore concluded that the observed effects were dependent on vasodilation by DA_1 stimulation and increased cardiac contractility by β_1-receptor stimulation, without any contribution from DA_2 receptors (15). In contrast, decrease of

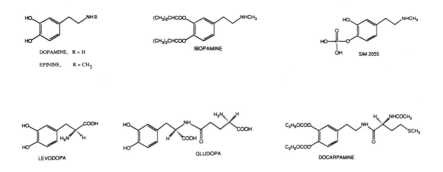

FIG. 2 - Formulae of dopamine prodrugs.

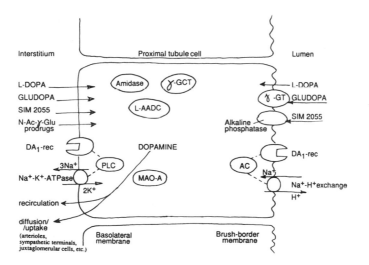

FIG. 3 - Transport and activation of dopamine prodrugs in proximal tubular cells.
L-AADC: L-aminoacid decarboxylase; γ-GT: γ-glutamyl transpeptidase; γ-GCT:
γ-glutamyl cyclotransferase; PLC : phospholipase C; AC: adenylate cyclase.

arterial NE was observed on acute administration by De Marco et al. (16).

Unfortunately, the effects on renal function were not assessed in these studies.

They deserve investigation in view of the active transport of endogenous levodo-

pa and local conversion into DA by dopadecarboxylase (L-amino acid decarboxy-

lase) in proximal tubular cells, as shown in Fig. 3, which also outlines the mecha-

nisms of transport and activation which can be exploited in the design of kidney-

selective prodrugs.

GLUDOPA

Gludopa was investigated as a development of the concept of renal target-

ing of drugs by conversion into γ-glutamyl derivatives, preferentially cleaved by

the highly concentrated γ-glutamyl transpeptidase of the brush border membrane

of the tubular cells (17) (Fig. 3). A different picture of the mechanisms underly-

ing the selectivity of these prodrugs has later been suggested from the investiga-

tion of the N-acetyl-γ-glutamyl prodrug of CGG 18137, a hydralazine-like vasod-

ilator (18). Active uptake by the organic anion transport system, which can also

transport levodopa and Sim 2055, or by a glutathione transport system is consid-

ered as the main determinant. Furthermore, cleavage by cytosolic γ-glutamyl

cyclotransferase would prevail on γ-glutamyl transpeptidase, being preceded by

deacetylation by an amidase in the case of the N-acetyl derivatives. Animal

studies showed that gludopa has selective renal effects and prevents acute renal

failure (4). Notwithstanding the lack of oral absorption, it was used by Lee and

associates as a tool in clinical investigations of the hypothesis that a fault of DA

mobilization in the kidney has a causative role in the development of essential

hypertension (19, 4). Infusion rates ranging from 12.5 to 100 µg/kg min induced

effects on RPF and Na$^+$ excretion comparable to 2 µg/kg min of DA, without any modification of systemic hemodynamics. Interestingly levodopa tended to lower PRA (20), at differences from fenoldopam; this was interpreted as a contribution of DA_2 mediated-mechanisms, suggesting that balanced stimulation of DA_1 and DA_2 receptors is a preferable approach to the treatment of hypertension, in comparison to selective stimulation of the DA_1 receptor. The latter has been shown to induce tolerance rapidly, because of direct stimulation of renin release and of reflex sympathetic activation. Although therapeutic applications of gludopa appear precluded, the supportive evidence provided by these studies to the perspective of orally active DA prodrugs as a treatment of hypertension is considerable.

Sim 2055

Sim 2055, i.e., epinine 4-O-phosphate, is a member of a series phosphate esters and diesters of catecholamines, depending for activation on hydrolysis by phosphatases and phosphodiesterases (21). Its diuretic and natriuretic effects in rats were comparable to those of IBO. In organ homogenates its rate of hydrolysis to epinine was proportional to alkaline phosphatase concentration, being maximal in the kidney and in the duodenum. It was well absorbed and metabolized in dogs, 70% of the dose being recovered in the 24 h urine as epinine sulphate conjugates, DOPAC and HVA; 2.8% of the dose was recovered as unmodified prodrugs (21). Hemodynamic investigations in anesthetized dogs showed that in the range from 1.25 to 10 mg/kg Sim 2055 induced a dose-dependent renal vasodilation, with no change in other parameters. In conscious dogs the renal hemodynamic effect of 0.625 - 2.5 mg/kg was comparable to an infusion of DA at 2-4 µg/kg/min (22). The selectivity of Sim 2055 can be referred to its activation by alkaline phosphatase; active uptake into the tubular cells, as shown in Fig. 3, as well as retention of epinine in these and other kidney cells can also contribute.

Sim 2055 chronically administered at 1-3 mg/kg p.o. bid for three months in two-clips two-kidneys hypertensive dogs significantly decreased systolic blood pressure. The effect lasted several hours after each dose, and was maintained over the treatment period (23). The suggestion has been advanced that Sim 2055 may elicit some direct action, owing to its prompt, DA-like effect on isolated organs, but the possibility that it may be due to a degree of hydrolysis in the organ preparation could not be discarded (24). It is interesting to recall the hypothesis that DA-3-O- and/or 4-O-phosphate may be present in the body and elicit a physiological role (25). Although clear evidence has not been produced to support this hypothesis, it has been shown that exogenous DA added to brain and salivary glands homogenates is in part converted to DA O-phosphates (26). Some kind of interaction of DA and the phosphate anion in the kidney is also suggested by the phosphaturia induced by DA and levodopa in dogs (27).

Clinical pharmacology study of Sim 2055 are now in progress in order to extend to humans the above observations.

CONCLUSIONS

The clinical use of ibopamine and the results obtained with other prodrugs, taken together with the important advancements of peripheral dopamine physiology and pharmacology, reinforce the promise of orally absorbed, kidney selective prodrugs, acting on both DA_1 and DA_2 receptors, in the therapy of congestive heart failure, and also of hypertension and chronic renal failure, and prompt further research in the field.

REFERENCES

1] McDonald, R.H. Jr., Goldberg, L.I., McNay, J.L., Tuttle, E.P. Effects of dopamine in man: augmentation of sodium excretion, glomerular filtration rate, and renal plasma flow. J Clin Invest. 1963; 43: 1116-1124

2] Felder, R.A., Carey, R.M., Eds., Proceedings of Third International Conference on Peripheral Dopamine. Am J Hypertens. 1990; 3 (Suppl)

3] Sibley, D.R., Monsma, F.J. Jr. Molecular biology of dopamine receptors. Trends Pharmacol Sci. 1992; 13: 61-69

4] Casagrande, C., Santangelo, F., in: Peripheral Dopamine Pathophysiology, Amenta F. Ed. CRC Press, Boca Raton, 1990; 307-343

5] Stella, V.J., Himmelstein, K.J. Prodrugs and site-specific drug delivery. J Med Chem. 1980; 23: 1275-1282

6] Smits, J.F., Thijssen, H.H. Spatial control of drug action: theoretical consideration on the pharmacokinetics of target-aimed drug delivery. In: Rate Controlled Drug Administration and Action, Struyker-Boudier, H. Ed., CRC Press, Boca Raton. 1986; 83-113

7] Godfraind, T., Spano, P.F., Carruba, M.O., Casagrande, C. Eds. Inodilators: a new strategy in the therapy of heart failure. J Cardiov Pharmacol. 1990; 14: (Suppl. 8)

8] Alleori, S., Beneduce, E., Scoppio, M., D'Agostino, A., Mele, G. The effects of ibopamine on peripheral vascular disease. Curr Ther Res. 1987; 42: 633-639

9] Docci, D., Pistocchi, E., Turci, F., Baldrati, L. Effect of ibopamine on the progression of chronic renal failure. Clin Nephrol. 1986; 26:121-124

10] Nishiyama, S., Yamaguchi, I., Akimoto, Y., Yoshikawa, M., Nakajima, H. A novel orally active dopamine prodrug TA-870. III. Positive inotropic effect and cardiorenal selectivity in anesthetized dogs. J Cardiovasc Pharmacol. 1990; 15: 283-290

11] Yoshikawa, M., Endo, H., Komatsu, K:, Fujihara, M., Takaiti, O., Kagoshima, T., Umehara, M., Ishikawa, H. Disposition of a new orally active dopamine prodrug, TA-870, in humans. Drug Met and Disp. 1990; 18: 212

12] Nishizaki, S., Fukuma A., Ogurusu, C., Hioka, T., Masaoka, Y., Takioka, M., Mikouchi, H., Nishizaki, Y. Acute effects of an orally active dopamine prodrug (TA-870) on systemic haemodynamics and renal functions. Drug Invest J. 1991; 3: 118-125

13] Kubota, J., Kubo, S., Nishimura, H., Ueyama, M., Kino, M., Nakayama, A., Hara, M., Kawamura, K. Cardiorenal effects of an orally active dopamine prodrug (TA-870) in patients with congestive heart failure. J Cardiov Pharmacol. 1989; 14: 53-57

14] Rajfer, S.I., Anton, A.H., Rossen, J.D., Goldberg, L.I. Beneficial hemodynamic effects of oral levodopa in heart failure. N Engl J Med., 1984; 310: 1357-1362

15] Rajfer, S.I., Rossen, J.D., Nemanich, J.W. Sustained hemodynamic improvement during long-term therapy with levodopa in heart failure. J Am Coll Cardiol. 1987; 10: 1286-1293

16] De Marco, T., Daly, P., Chatterjee, K. Systemic and coronary hemodynamic and neurohumoral effects of levodopa in congestive heart failure. Am J Cardiol. 1988; 62: 1228-1233

17] Magnan, S.D.J., Shirota, F.N., Nagasawa, H.T. Drug latentiation by γ-glutamyl transpeptidase. J Med Chem. 1982; 25: 1018-1021

18] Drieman, J.C., Thijssen, H.H.W., Zeegers, H.H.M., Smits, J.F.M., Struyker Boudier, H.A.J. Renal selective N-acetyl-γ-glutamyl prodrugs: a study on the mechanism of activation of the renal vasodilator prodrug CGP 22979. Br J Pharmacol. 1990; 99: 15-20

19] Lee, M.R. Salt, renal dopamine and essential hypertension. Triangle 1987; 26: 11-22

20] Worth, D.P., Harvey, J.N., Brown, J., Worral, A., Lee, M.R. Domperidone treatment in man inhibits the fall in plasma renin activity induced by intravenous γ-L-glutamyl-L-dopa. J Clin Pharmacol. 1986; 21: 497-502

21] Casagrande, C., Merlo, L., Santangelo, F. N-methyldopamine 4-O-phosphate, an orally active renal vasodilator. 10th Int. Symp. Med. Chem., Budapest, 1988; Abs 87

22] Casagrande, C., Merlo, L., Ferrini, R., Miragoli, G., Semeraro, C. Cardiovascular and renal action of dopaminergic prodrugs. J Cardiov Pharmacol. 1989; 14: (Suppl) S40-S59

23] Semeraro, C., Casati, C., Merlo, L., Miragoli, G., Pradella, L., Pocchiari, F., Zambon, C. Antihypertensive effect of Sim 2055: a new renal selective dopaminergic agent. 4th International Conference on Peripheral Dopamine, Porto, 1992; P 27

24] Marchini, F., Ferlenga, P., Allievi, L., Pocchiari, F., Semeraro, C. In vitro metabolism and peripheral dopaminergic activity of Sim 2055, an epinine prodrug. 4th International Conference on Peripheral Dopamine, Porto, 1992; P 36

25] Byington, K.H. Pharmacological properties of a phosphate ester of dopamine. Life Science 1987; 40: 2091-2095

26] Byington, K.H. Biological phosphorylation of dopamine. FASEB J. 1992; 6: A1023

27] Cuche, J.L., Marchand, G.M., Greger, R.F., Lang, F.C., Knox, F.G. Phosphaturic effect of dopamine in dogs. Possible role of intrarenally produced dopamine in phosphate regulation. J Clin Invest 1976; 58: 71-76

ABSTRACTS

Renal metabolism of catecholamines in response to increased dietary phosphate intake.

G. M. Tyce T. J. Berndt, A. MacDonald, R. Walikonis, S. Chinnow, T. P. Dousa & F. G. Knox.
Department of Physiology and Biophysics, Mayo Graduate School of Medicine, Rochester, Minnesota, U.S.A.

The urinary excretion of free dopamine, norepinephrine, and epinephrine ,reflects the contribution of both the neural release of these catecholamines and intrarenal synthesis and metabolism of dopamine. Since these catecholamines are rapidly metabolized the excretion of the free amines represents only a fraction of the total release and synthesis by the kidney. The aim of the present study was to determine the effect of increasing dietary phosphate intake on the excretion of free dopamine norepinephrine, and epinephrine, and their primary stable metabolites. Seven male rats were placed in metabolic balance cages and fed 12 g/day of normal phosphate diet (0.7% Pi, NPD) for 4 days and then fed a high phosphate diet (1.8% Pi, HPD) for 4 days. Twenty-four hour urine samples were collected for determination of free dopamine, norepinephrine, epinephrine, their major stable metabolites, and electrolyte excretions. Concentrations of catecholamines were measured by HPLC with eletrochemical detection. The urinary excretion data for the seven rats was combined for all four days of NPD or HPD.

Increasing phosphate intake from 0.7% Pi to 1.8% Pi significantly increased phosphate and free dopamine excretion (5.9±0.4 to 6.8±0.1 μg/day, mean ± SEM). This increase in free dopamine excretion was associated with similar increases (when expressed as a percentage relative to NPD) in urinary excretion of dopamine metabolites, 3,4-dihydroxyphenylacetic acid, 8.9±0.4 to 12.1±0.6 μg/day and homovanillic acid, 17.2±0.6 to 21.3±0.7 μg/day. No change was noted in excretion of 3-methoxtyramine, the O-methylated metabolite of dopamine, or in dopamine sulfate in rats fed NPD or HPD. DOPA in plasma is considered to be the major source of urinary dopamine, but plasma DOPA was unchanged by increased phosphate intake. Excretions of free and sulfated norepinephrine or normetanephrine were not changed by increased phosphate intake. However, excretion of 3-methoxy-4-hydroxyphenylglycol, a major metabolite of norepinephrine and epinephrine, decreased signifcantly (34.9±1.5 to 24.1±0.7 μg/day). These observations demonstrated that urinary-free dopamine excretion represents a fraction of total dopamine synthesis and that increases in phosphate intake also result in a generalized increase in the excretion of several, but not all, of its major metabolites.

Effect of changes in dietary phosphate intake on urinary dopamine excretion.

T. J. Berndt, J. Isaac, T. P. Dousa, G. M. Tyce & F. G. Knox.
Department of Physiology and Biophysics, Mayo Graduate School of Medicine, Rochester, Minnesota, U.S.A.

Dopamine is synthesized by proximal tubules and has also been demonstrated to increase phosphate excretion. Studies were performed to determine the effect of changes in dietary phosphate intake on renal dopamine synthesis as reflected by 24-hour urinary excretion of dopamine. Seven male rats were placed in metabolic cages and fed 12 g/day of a normal phosphate diet (NPD, 0.7% Pi) for 4 days. Sodium, potassium, and chloride contents in NPD and LPD were made similar to HPD by adding sodium chloride and potassium carbonate to the food. Urine samples were collected for twenty-four hours for determination of free dopamine, norepinephrine, epinephrine, and electrolyte excretions. Concentrations of catecholamines were determined by HPLC with electrochemical detection.

Within the first twenty-four hours of selectively increasing phosphate intake from 0.7% Pi to 1.8% Pi, both phosphate excretion significantly increased from 1.8 ± 0.2 to 5.8 ± 0.2 mM/day, and free dopamine excretion signifcantly increased from 3.7 ± 0.3 to 5.2 ± 0.3 µg/day, without changes in sodium, cAMP, creatinine, norepinephrine or epinephrine excretions. Similarly; decreasing phosphate intake from 1.8% Pi to 0.07% Pi markedly decreased phosphate excretion from 5.3 ± 0.1 to 0.3 ± 0.02 mM/day, and free dopamine excretion from 4.0 ± 0.3 µg/day on the last day of HPD to 3.2 ± 0.1 µg/day within the first 24 hours of LPD ($P<0.05$).

These observations demonstrate that changes in dietary phosphate intake result in parallel changes in urinary dopamine and phosphate excretion. Additional studies demonstrated that infusion of dopamine to rats fed LPD (0.07% Pi) enhanced the phosphaturic effect of parathyroid hormone (PTH) in rats fed an LPD for 3 days. PTH (33 U/kg + 1 U/kg/min) had no effect on Pi excretion (FEpi 0.5 ± 0.2 - $0.3\pm0.1\%$, n=5) whereas in the presence of dopamine infusion (25 µg/kg/min), PTH significantly increased Pi excretion (FEpi 0.8 ± 0.4 - $11.5\pm1.7\%$, n=5). Dopamine also increased phosphate excretion in rats fed a low phosphate diet for 2 days (FEpi, 1.2 ± 0.07 - $12.0\pm2.9\%$, n=5), Thus, renal dopamine synthesis responds to changes in the dietary intake of Pi and, when administered exogenously, can override the Pi retaining effects of Pi deprivation.

Is dopamine an intrarenal hormone? Re-examination of the question based on in vitro studies with renal epithelial cells.

Dennis P. Healy & Arcady Grenader.
Depanment of Pharmacology, Mount Sinai School of Medicine, New York, NY.

Studies with whole animals have demonstrated that: 1) exogenously administered dopamine (DA) is a potent natriuretic/diuretic agent, 2) sodium loading increases urinary excretion of DA, and 3) saline-induced natriuresis can be blocked by inhibition of DA synthesis or DA receptor blockade. These findings have led to the hypothesis that DA is an intrarenal natriuretic hormone. We sought to determine whether evidence in support of this hypothesis could be obtained in vitro. Using cultured renal epithelial cells, we examined: 1) whether renal cells could produce DA from L-dopa, and 2) whether locally formed DA could stimulate DA receptors in an autocrine/paracrine manner. The proximal tubule-like epithelial cell line, LLC-PK1 expresses a high affinity DA1 receptor that stimulates adenylyl cyclase activity. We determined that LLC-PK1 cells contained high levels of the aromatic L-amino acid decarboxylase (AADC). Incubation of LLC-P1 cells with L-dopa resulted in formation of DA and its secretion into the media effects that were blocked by AADC inhibitors. L-Dopa also stimulated cAMP accumulation in the LLC-PK1 cells, effects that were blocked by D_1 receptor antagonists or inhibitors of AADC.

Inner medullary collecting duct (IMCD) cells express high levels of a D_2-like receptor, termed D_{2K}. Activation of the D_{2K} receptor results in increased production of prostaglandin E_2 (PGE_2). IMCD cells contained significant levels of AADC, although much less than in LLC-PK1 cells. Incubation of IMCD cells with L-dopa resulted in formation of DA and stimulation of PGE_2 production eflects that were blocked by AADC inhibition or D_2 antagonists. AADC inhibitors and D_2 antagonists lowered basal PGE_2 levels suggesting that DA was being constitutively produced and released by IMCD cells.

These results indicate that renal epithelial cells can produce DA intracellularly by uptake and enzymatic conversion of L-DOPA. The locally formed DA is rapidly secreted and stimulates cell-surface DA receptors. These findings are consistent with DA being an autocrine/paracrine agent in renal epithelial cells and therefore provide support for the hypothesis that DA is an intrarenal hormone.

Dopamine production in rat isolated renal tubular epithelial cells.

J.T. Guimarães* & P.Soares-da-Silva.
Dept. of Pharmacology & Therapeutics, Faculty of Medicine, 4200 Porto, Portugal.

There is evidence suggesting that dopamine (DA) formed within tubular epithelial cells may act as an autocrine and/or paracrine substance in the regulation of sodium reabsorption through the activation of specific tubular D_1 receptors. The aim of the present work was to study the formation of DA in isolated renal tubular epithelial cells and to seek further information on the processes interfering with the regulation of dopamine synthesis. Tubular epithelial cells were obtained from rat renal cortex; the tissues were minced to a paste like consistency, incubated with collagenase (0.06%) and thereafter poured through graded sieves (180, 75, 53 and 23 µm) to obtain a single cell suspension. The viability of the cells, tested under light microscopy after the addition of trypan blue, was about 80%. Isolated cells were handled in Dulbecco's Modified Eagle (DME) medium or Hank's medium and the experiments on the synthesis of DA were carried out at 25° C in an atmosphere of 95% O_2 and 5% CO_2. The cell suspension was preincubated for 15 min, in a water shaking bath, and thereafter incubated with increasing concentrations of L-DOPA (1 to 500 µM) for further 15 min; in some experiments, the cell suspension was incubated with 50 µM L-DOPA for increasing periods of time (1 to 15 min). The time-dependent (1 to 15min) formation of DA and DOPAC in the presence of 50 µM L-DOPA was found to be greater in experiments using the Hank's medium (DA, 3.3±0.2 to 36.0±4.3 nmol/mg protein; DOPAC, 2.0±0.8 to 11.7±2.0 nmol/mg protein) than when using DME medium (DA, 1.9±0.7 to 16.5±2.7 nmol/mg protein; DOPAC, 0.2±0.1 to 2.8±0.1 nmol/mg protein). The concentration-dependent (1 to 500 µM L-DOPA) formation of DA and DOPAC during 15 min incubation period was also found to be greater in experiments using the Hank's medium (DA, 1.6±0.2 to 70.3±8.8 nmol/mg protein; DOPAC, 0.4±0.4 to 8.5±2.8 nmol/mg protein) than when using DME medium (DA, 0.5±0.2 to 65.4±7.6 nmol/mg protein; DOPAC, 0.3±0.04 to 11.1±1.4 nmol/mg protein). Inhibition of Na^+-K^+ ATPase with ouabain (1 and 2 mM) or an excess of potassium (45 and 90 mM) did not modify the concentration- and time-dependent pattern of amine formation. In contrast to that obtained in kidney slices (1), the formation of DA in isolated tubular cells incubated in DME medium was found not to be affected by the inhibition of Na^+-K^+ ATPase. These results show that freshly obtained tubular cells are a feasible preparation to study the synthesis of DA, though DME medium may be not the best incubation medium to perform such studies.

(1) Soares-da-Silva P, Fernandes M.H. Br.J.Pharmacol., 105:811-816,1992.
Supported by INIC (FmP1).
*on leave from the Dept. of Biochemistry, Fac. Medicine, 4200 Porto, Portugal.

Peripheral dopamine, its precursors and metabolites in human aging.

Otto Kuchel
Clinical Research Institute of Montreal, Hôtel-Dieu of Montreal Hospital and University of Montreal, Montreal, Quebec, CANADA.

While human aging is known to be associated with an increased plasma norepinephrine (NE) due to its increased appearance, there are only few data on the effect of aging on peripheral dopamine (DA) and its metabolites, and even less on the DA precursors dihydroxyphenylalanine (DOPA) and tyrosine.

We compared indices of DA, DOPA and tyrosine release and the tyrosine suppressibility by DOPA in healthy subjects of a young (mean age 25) and older (mean age 52) age group prior to and after a single L-DOPA (500 mg) administration. Under baseline conditions, older subjects compared to younger ones had lower ($P<0.05$) plasma levels of 3-0-methylDOPA (a main DOPA metabolite and its marker), a higher ($P<0.05$) plasma tyrosine:DOPA ratio (suggesting a higher tyrosine supply but lower neuronal DOPA release), higher ($P<0.05$) urinary excretions of two main NE metabolites (normetanephrine and NE sulfate) but lower ($P<0.05$) urinary dihydroxyphenylacetic acid (DOPAC) excretion. Following L-DOPA administration, older subjects had a lower ($P<0.05$) plasma tyrosine suppressibility, more ($P<0.05$) plasma free DA increase but a lower ($P<0.05$) rise in plasma and urinary DOPAC (a marker of the intraneuronal deamination of DA), a lower ($P<0.05$) rise in plasma homovanillic acid and a lower ($P<0.05$) rise in the glomerular DOPA load. The increase in urinary DA and DOPAC excretions was also lower ($P<0.05$).

In conclusion, the overall higher NE appearance in older subjects (an almost unanimous finding in the literature) appears to be driven by a higher appearance of the NE precursor DA which is probably rather taken up by the vesicles to generate NE than intraneuronally deaminated to DOPAC. Older subjects probably have also a higher supply of the DA precursor DOPA at the expense of the neuronal release of DOPA, plasma DOPA concentration and glomerular DOPA load, the latter resulting in an impairment of the renal DA formation. Finally, older subjects appear to have a higher supply of tyrosine, the ultimate catecholamine precursor.

(Supported by the Medical Research Council of Canada).

Ontogeny of the renal tubular dopamine synthetising and cellular transport systems in dog.

P.Soares-da-Silva, M.H.Fernandes, M.Pestana, M.A.Vieira-Coelho & J.T.Guimarães.
Dept. of Pharmacology & Therapeutics, Faculty of Medicine, 4200 Porto, Portugal.

There is evidence in the literature that maturation of renal functions is a slow development process and newborn subjects may have a deffective control in the renal handling of water and electrolytes. Dopamine is a natriuretic hormone which can be produced within the kidney, namely in tubular epithelial cells from dihydroxylphenylalanine (DOPA) present in the tubular filtrate. The aim of the present work was, therefore, to evaluate the ability of renal tissues of developing animals to synthesize dopamine and the cell outward transport of the amine. Renal tissues from newborn dogs (less than 24 hours after birth), 10 days and 2 months aged dogs and adult animals were used. In some experiments, renal cortical slices were incubated for 15 min with increasing concentrations of L-DOPA (5 to 5000 μM) and the amounts of DA and its deaminated metabolite DOPAC determined; DA and DOPAC levels were determined both in kidney slices and the incubation medium, in order to allow the determination of the fractional outflow of the two compounds. In other experiments, kidney homogenates were used and the kinetics of the enzyme aromatic L-amino acid decarboxylase (AAAD) determined. The formation of DA and DOPAC in kidney slices was found to be dependent on the concentration of L-DOPA added to the medium and saturable at 5000 μM L-DOPA; the synthesis of DA and its deamination to DOPAC was, however, found to be in adult dogs 2.5-fold that in 2 months aged dogs, 3.1-fold that in 10 days aged dogs and 13-fold that in newborn animals. The kinetics (V_{max}, in pmol/mg protein/h; K_m, in μM) of the AAAD determined in kidney homogenates were as follows: adults ($V_{max}=3583\pm345$; $K_m=181\pm23$), 2 months aged ($V_{max}=1169\pm112$; $K_m=244\pm19$), 10 days aged ($V_{max}=685\pm75$; $K_m=190\pm12$) and newborn ($V_{max}=247\pm25$; $K_m=80\pm5$). The V_{max} for the outward cell transfer of DA was in adult dogs of 112 ± 16 nmol/g/15 min and significantly lower in the 2 months aged (19 ± 5 nmol/g/15 min), 10 days aged (25 ± 3 nmol/g/15 min) and in newborn dogs (6.0 ± 1.4 nmol/g/15 min). It is concluded that, in the dog, maturation of the DA synthetising and cell outward amine transfer systems are slowly developing processes.

Supported by INIC (FmP1).

Quantitative difference of regional dopamine generation from 3,4-dihydroxyphenylalanine (DOPA) in the peripheral tissues.

Shuichi Shigetomi, Kiyonobu Tanaka, Jin-chi Kim &Soitsu Fukuchi.
Internal Medicine III, Fukushima Medical College, Fukushima-City, JAPAN 960-12

Aromatic L-amino acid decarboxylase (AAAD) catalyzing the conversion of L-DOPA to dopamine (DA) exists universally in the peripheral tissues. DA generated in the periphery is known to be a paracrine hormone and exhibits its physiolngical action by stimulating nearby DA receptors. In the present study, we demonstrated the distribution of L-DOPA and the DA gencration and metabolism in the peripheral tissues following exogenous L-DOPA administration. **Methods**: Twenty-four male Sprague-Dawley rats were used. After measuring basal blood pressure (BP), L-DOPA (l00 mg/kg) was administered intraperitoneally and rats were killed by decapitation 30, 60 and 120 minutes after the administration. Tissues (kidney, liver, adrenal gland, lung and skeletal muscle) were removed and the contents of L-DOPA, 3,4-dihydroxyphenylacetic acid (DOPAC) , homovanillic acid (HVA), 3-methoxytyramine (3-MT), norepinephrine and epinephrine were measured by HPLC with electrochemical detection. **Results**: L-DOPA induced a slight decrease in BP. Basal L-DOPA contents of the tissues were comparable (1-3 nmol/g tissue). 30 minutes after the administration, L-DOPA contents markedly increase in all tissues. The accumulation of L-DOPA in the skeletal muscle was the greatest (100-fold increase of the initial). DA in the renal cortex and medulla considerably increased (cortex: control 0.6 ± 0.6, 30 min 169 ± 54 nmol/g tissue and medulla: control 0.03 ± 0.03, 30 min 118 ± 104 nmol/g tissue) accompanied by the concomitant increases in DOPAC, HVA and 3-MT. DA also increased in other tissues; liver (0.03 ± 0.02 to 19 ± 12 nmol/g tissue), lung (0.009 ± 0.004 to 6.5 ± 1.8 nmol/g tissue) and skeletal muscle (0.08 ± 0 0.8 to 0.8 ± 0.3 nmol/g tissue), but not in the adrenal gland (3.0 ± 2.3 to 1.7 ± 1.5 mmol/g tissue). The ratio of L-DOPA to DA was significantly lower in the renal cortex and medulla than those of the other tissues, while the ratio of the skeletal muscle was the highest of all. **Conclusions**: These results suggest that the peripheral DA generation is quantitattvely different among the tissues, and that the kidney is a predominant organ producing DA from L-DOPA. The skeletal muscle may become a reservoir of L-DOPA when plasma L-DOPA level is elevated.

© 1993 Pergamon Press Ltd.
Printed in Great Britain.

Preferential decarboxylation of L-*threo*-DOPS in renal tissues.

P.Soares-da-Silva.
Dept. of Pharmacology & Therapeutics, Faculty of Medicine, 4200 Porto, Portugal.

L-*threo*-dihydroxyphenylserine (L-*threo*-DOPS) has long been shown to be unique among the available precursors of catecholamines; it undergoes direct conversion into natural (-)-noradrenaline by the action of the enzyme aromatic L-amino acid decarboxylase (AAAD). Administration of L-*threo*-DOPS has been reported to increase tissue and plasma levels of noradrenaline and to improve orthostatic hypotension, by rising blood pressure, in several pathological conditions, namely in patients with deficiency of dopamine ß-hydroxylase. The rise in blood pressure, however, as induced by L-*threo*-DOPS has been demonstrated to be similar in control and denervated animals, introducing the possibility of a major role of non-neuronal AAAD. The aim of the present work was, therefore, to study the formation of noradrenaline in several peripheral tissues particularly rich in non-neuronal AAAD activity (renal cortex, jejunum and liver) and the left ventricle, in which AAAD activity appears to be confined to sympathetic nerves. Male Wistar rats (200-240 g weight) were given L-*threo*-DOPS (3, 10 or 30 mg/kg, i.p.) and sacrificed 15 min after the injection. In other experiments, animals were given L-*threo*-DOPS (10 mg/kg, i.p.) and sacrificed 5, 15, 30, 60 or 90 min after the injection. The accumulation of newly-formed noradrenaline in the jejunum, liver and renal cortex was found to be dependent on the dose of L-*threo*-DOPS given, whereas in the left ventricle at the dose of 30 mg/kg L-*threo*-DOPS the tissue levels of noradrenaline were even lower than those observed at 3 and 10 mg/kg. At 30 mg/kg L-*threo*-DOPS the tissue levels of noradrenaline increased by 21-fold in the renal cortex, 4.4-fold in the liver and 2.8-fold in the jejunum; in the left ventricle, the tissue levels of noradrenaline after 3 and 10 mg/kg L-*threo*-DOPS increased by 56% and 50%, respectively. The accumulation of noradrenaline after the administration of L-*threo*-DOPS was also a time-dependent effect, reaching its maximum at 15 min and then declining progressively. The accumulation of 3,4-dihydroxyphenylglycol (DOPEG), the deaminated metabolite of noradrenaline, followed that of its parent amine. Pretreatment with benserazide (6.8 mg/kg, i.p.) completely abolished the formation of noradrenaline in rats given 30 mg/kg L-*threo*-DOPS. Denervation by 6-OHDA did not affect the formation of noradrenline in the renal cortex, liver and jejunum of rats given L-*threo*-DOPS (30 mg/kg). It is concluded that renal tissues preferentially decarboxylate L-*threo*-DOPS into noradrenaline, followed by the liver and jejunum, and non-neuronal AAAD has a major role in this process.

Supported by a grant from the INIC.

Evaluation of the dopamine synthetising systems in the rat digestive tract.

M.A. Vieira-Coelho & P.Soares-da-Silva.
Dept. of Pharmacology & Therapeutics, Faculty of Medicine, 4200 Porto, Portugal.

Epithelial cells of renal tubules, namely those of the proximal portion of the nephron, are endowed with a great aromatic L-amino acid decarboxylase activity (AAAD). These cells synthesize dopamine from dihydroxyphenylalanine (DOPA) present in the tubular filtrate and the amine thus formed has been shown of importance in the renal handling of water and electrolytes. The intestine, namely its duodenal and ileal portions, have also been shown to possess high amounts of the enzyme AAAD and there is evidence to suggest that locally formed dopamine may be implicated in the regulation of sodium and water absorption in this organ. The aim of the present work was to study the formation of dopamine along the rat digestive tract under in vitro experimental conditions; the deamination of dopamine into 3,4-dihydroxyphenylacetic acid (DOPAC) was also studied. The assay of dopamine and DOPAC was performed by means of h.p.l.c. with electrochemical detection. The selected tissues were the non-glandular stomach, duodenum, jejunum, ileum and proximal and distal colon. In some experiments, tissues were incubated with 500 µM L-DOPA for 20 min in conditions of COMT inhibition (50 µM tropolone); the formation of dopamine was found to be in the duodenum, jejunum and ileum 2-fold that in the proximal colon and 115-fold that in the non-glandular stomach and the distal colon. The accumulation of DOPAC in these tissues followed that of the parent amine. The formation of dopamine in jejunal segments loaded with L-DOPA was found to be dependent on the concentration of L-DOPA (50 to 5000 µM) used. Because of limited solubility of L-DOPA, saturation of the decarboxylation could not be achieved. On the other hand, the formation of DOPAC was saturable at 1000 µM L-DOPA (corresponding to 600 nmol/g of dopamine). In another set of experiments, it was found that in jejunal segments loaded with increasing concentrations of L-DOPA (50, 100 and 500 µM) the formation of dopamine was dependent on the time of incubation. The rate constant (k) of formation of dopamine as a function of time was found to be similar (0.050 ± 0.005) with either concentration of L-DOPA, whereas the rate constant of DOPAC formation was greater at the highest concentrations of L-DOPA. These results show that the formation of dopamine from L-DOPA along the digestive tract presents an heterogeneous pattern, being the small intestine and the proximal colon the areas where this reaction appears to be more important. It is also shown that the jejunal transport system of L-DOPA into the compartment where the synthesis takes place is not saturable up to 5 mM L-DOPA.

Supported by a grant from the INIC.

Renal outflow of dopamine: A comparative study in human and rat renal tissues.

M. Pestana & P. Soares-da-Silva.
Dept. of Pharmacology & Therapeutics, Faculty of Medicine , 4200 Porto, Portugal.

There is evidence that the endogenous dopamine (DA) may act as an autocrine and/or paracrine substance reducing sodium reabsorption through the activation of specific renal tubular D_1 receptors. Renal tissues are endowed with one of the highest monoamine oxidase (MAO) activities in the body and deamination of newly-formed DA into 3,4-dihydroxyphenylacetic acid (DOPAC) represents a major pathway for the inactivation of the amine. Information is lacking, however, on the mechanisms which regulate the fate and outflow of newly-formed DA and DOPAC in tubular epithelial cells. The aim of the present work was, therefore, to perform a comparative study of the outflow of newly-formed DA and DOPAC in human (n=4) and rat (n=4) renal tissues previously loaded with exogenous L-DOPA (100 µM); tissues were perifused with warm (37°C) and gassed (95% O_2 and 5% CO_2) Krebs solution; after stabilization, five consecutive 10 min fractions of the perifusate were collected. DA and DOPAC levels in the perifusate (in nmol/g/10 min) were logarithmicaly transformed, plotted against time of perifusion and the constant rates of outflow for the amine and its deaminated metabolite calculated; the fractional outflow and the tissue levels of DA and DOPAC at the end of the perifusion period were also determined. The levels of DA and DOPAC in the outflow progressively declined with similar constant rates of loss while using either human or rat renal tissues (0.0388±.0021 vs 0.0372±0.0015); in both series the fractional outflow of DOPAC was significantly higher than that for DA. In addition, while using human renal fragments DA levels were significantly lower than those found in the rat, either in tissues (0.80±0.12 nmol/g vs 4.98±0.61 nmol/g) and the perifusate (0.28 to 0.06 nmol/g/10 min vs 1.10 to 0.25 nmol/g/10 min); by contrast, the DOPAC levels were similar in human and rat tissues (1.90±0.61 vs 1.67±0.31 nmol/g), being DOPAC levels in the perifusate of the human kidney significantly higher than that in the rat (2.25 to 0.37 vs 0.91 to 0.27 nmol/g/10 min); this results in higher DOPAC/DA ratios in tissue (2.65±0.92 vs 0.33±0.04) and perifusate samples (14±5 vs 1±0.15) of experiments using human tissues. These results suggest that the kinetic characteristics of the efflux of DA and DOPAC are similar in both human and rat renal tissues and also show that the fraction of newly-formed DA which is leaving the tubular cells is a constant source for DOPAC. Evidence favouring the view that deamination of DA is more intense in human tissues was also obtained; this agrees with different deamination activities in human and rat renal tissues.

Supported by a grant from the INIC (FmP1).

Dopamine effects in Dahl salt-sensitive rats.

Anita Aperia, Akinori Nishi, Alejandro Bertorello, Ann-Christine Eklöf & Gianni Celsi.
Dept. Pediatrics, Karolinska Institutet, St. Göran's Children's Hospital, Stockholm, Sweden.

The kidney fluid system is responsible for the longterm control of blood pressure. The renal salt excretion is related to blood pressure in such a way that the pressure rarely deviates more than 10%. In hypertension, the relationship between pressure and salt excretion is altered. It has been suggested that altered function of factors regulating renal sodium transport are the cause of salt-sensirive hypertension. Dopamine (DA) is produced in renal proximal tubule cells, and is a natriuretic hormone that acts by inhibiting the activity of $Na^+,K^+ATPase$. $Na^+,K^+ATPase$ activity is inhibited in the proximal tubule (PT) by a synergistic action of D_1 and D_2 receptors and in the thick ascending limb of Henle (TAL) by activation of the D_1 receptor only. During high salt intake, $Na^+,K^+ATPase$ activity is downregulated by dopamine. Renal dopamine production is increased and the sensitivity to dopamine might be enhanced.

We now show, using Dahl salt-sensitive and salt-resistent rats on normal salt diet, that the effect of dopamine on renal sodium excretion and on $Na^+,K^+ATPase$ activity in PT and TAL is blunted in Dahl salt sensitive rats. $Na^+,K^+ATPase$ activity is not downregulated during high salt diet. High salt diet causes a paradoxical increase in mRNA for both $Na^+,K^+ATPase$ subunits, indicating increased enzyme turnover. We interpret the lack of effect of dopamine to be due to a defect coupling between the D_1 receptor and the adenylate cyclase unit, since both DA and D_1 agonist, fenoldopam failed to increase cAMP levels in cortical and outer medullary tubules. The lack of effect of DA on renal tubule $Na^+,K^+ATPase$ activity and the lack of natriuretic response to DA is present before hypertension is induced by high salt diet.

Conclusion. Dopamine regulation of renal sodium transport is, due to defect coupling between the D_1 receptor and adenylate cyclase, blunted in Dahl salt-sensitive rats. This defect which precedes the development of hypertension, might conbribute to altered blood pressure regulation in Dahl salt-sensitive rats.

© 1993 Pergamon Press Ltd.
Printed in Great Britain.

Dopamine receptor blockade and synthesis inhibition during exaggerated natriuresis in spontaneously hypertensive rats.

Peter Hansell & Mats Sjöqvist.
Dept. of Physiology, Biomedical Center, University of Uppsala, Sweden

The influence of dopamine receptor blockade and synthesis inhibition on natriuresis induced by isotonic saline volume expansion was investigated in anaesthetized spontaneously hypertensive rats (SHR) and normotensive Wistar-Kyoto rats (WKY). The aim of the study was to elucidate the mechanisms underlying the phenomenon of exaggerated natriuresis during volume expansion that has been observed in SHR.

Volume expansion, at 5 % of body weight, resulted in a larger and faster natriuretic response in SHR than in WKY. Sixty minutes after commencement of volume expansion the natriuretic response (accumulated sodium excretion) in WKY (n=8, 88±25 μmoles) was only 24 % of that in SHR (n=17, 362±58 μmoles). Compared with vehicle-treated SHR the natriuetic response to volume expansion was only 16 % and 35 % in SHR-animals pretreated with the dopamine receptor blockers haloperidol (n=14, 1 mg.kg^{-1}) and SCH23390 (n=8, 30 μg.kg^{-1}) , respectively, and only 59 % and 42 % when pretreated with the dopamine synthesis inhibitor benserazide at two different doses (n=8, 50 mg.kg^{-1}; n=5, 100 mg.kg^{-1}). The corresponding proportion in haloperidol-treated (n=8) compared with vehicle-treated WKY rats was 22 %.

In conclusion, isotonic volume loading results in more pronounced natriuresis in SHR than in WKY. Dopamine receptor blockade and synthesis inhibition attenuate the exaggerated natriuresis in SHR and reduces the VE-induced natriuresis in WKY. The results indicate that the dopamine-system plays an important role in the natriuretic response to saline volume loading in both SHR and WKY and accounts for a major part of the exaggerated natriuresis in SHR.

© 1993 Pergamon Press Ltd.
Printed in Great Britain.

Pharmacological characterization of dopamine D_1 receptor binding sites in human circulating mononuclear cells.

F. Veglio, G. Pinna, A. Ricci*, M- Ruffa, D. Schiavone & F. Amenta*
Cattedra Medicina Interna Universi di Torino Osp. S. Vito, Torino and *Dip. to Sanità Pubblica e Biologia Cellulare, Università "Tor Vergata", Roma, Italy.

Circulating blood cells are rich in neurotransmitter receptors. The significance of neurotransmitter receptors on blood cells is not well understood. However their analysis offer a good opportunity to study disease- or drug-induced alterations of a given receptor population.

The present study was designed to investigate the characteristics of dopamine D_1 receptors in preparations of human circulating mononuclear cells in normotensive and essential hypertensive patients using radioligand binding techniques. ^{3}H-SCH 23390 was used as a label of these receptors.

In normotensive subjects ^{3}H-SCH 23390 was bound to circulating mononuclear cells in a manner consistent with the labelling of dopamine D_1 receptors. The dissociation constant (K_d) value was 0.8 nM and the maximum density of binding sites (B_{max}) was 285±15 fmol/10 cells. The B_{max} value was significantly reduced in hypertensive subjects whereas the K_d did not change.

Further studies are in progress to evaluate whether the binding sites identified in the present study fulfill the criteria to be considered dopamine D_1 receptors.

Autoradiographic localization of [3H]-dopexamine in the human heart.

P. Napoleone, A. Ricci * & F. Amenta
Dipto di Sanità Pubblica e Biologia Cellulare, Università "Tor Vergata" and * Dipto di Scienze Cardiovascolari e Respiratorie Università "La Sapienza", Roma (Italy).

Dopexamine hydrochloride (DPX) is a structural analogue of dopamine, acting as an agonist on peripheral dopamine D_1 and D_2 receptors as well as $ß_2$-adreneceptors, proposed primarily for the short-term treatment of acute heart failure.

In the present study we investigated, using radioreceptor binding and autoradiographic techniques, the pharmacological features and the anatomical localization of [3H]-DPX binding to sections of human heart. Specimens of ventricles were obtained from heart removed to be transplanted and then found not suitable for transplantation due to the presence of traumatic lesions.

[3H]-DPX binding to sections of ventricles was time-, temperature- and concentration-dependent. Incubation of sections in the presence of specific $ß_2$-adrenoceptor or dopamine receptor antagonists demonstrated that [3H]-DPX labeled both $ß_2$-adrenoceptors and D_2 receptors while no binding to D_1 sites occurred in human heart. Autoradiography revealed the presence of [3H]-DPX binding sites throughout the ventricular wall, with a slight prevalence in the right ventricle. [3H]-DPX binding sites were located primarily within myocytes. No difference in the density of binding sites was noticeable along the thickness of the ventricular wall. Incubation in the presence of specific antagonists revealed that $ß_2$-adrenoceptor blockade reduced [3H]-DPX binding sites density by about 80% and D_2 receptor blockade by about 20%.

These data may suggest that the cardiac effect of DPX discribed in humans are mediated through the interaction with $ß_2$-adrenoceptors and D_2 receptors located within the myocardial tissue.

Dopamine D_1 receptor sites in the human umbilical artery of normotensive and pre-eclamptic subjects: A radioligand and autoradiographic study.

J.A. Ferreira de Almeida[1], A. Ricci[2], L. Pereira Leite[1] & F. Amenta[2].
[1] Clinica Obstétrica, Faculdade de Medicina do Porto, Porto (Portugal).
[2] Dipto di Sanitá Pubblica e Biologia Cellulare, Università "Tor Vergata", Roma (Italy).

The pharmacological profile and the anatomical localization of dopamine D_1 receptor sites were analyzed in sections of the umbilical artery taken from normotensive and pre-eclamptic patients using radioligand binding and autoradiographic techniques respectively. [^{3}H]-SCH 23390 was used to label D_1 sites.

[^{3}H]-SCH 23390 was bound to sections of human umbilical artery in a manner consistent with the labeling of dopamine D_1 receptors in the normotensive and pre-eclamptic subjects. The density of dopamine D_1 receptors which is higher placental than in the fetal end was significantly reduced in pre-ealampsia. The decrease was more pronounced in the placental end.

Light microscope autoradiography revealed the accumulation of [^{3}H]-SCH 23390 within smooth muscle of the medial layer of umbilical arteries with a fetal-to-maternal gradient. Consistent with radioligand binding experiments, a loss of [^{3}H]-SCH 23390 binding sites, was noticeable in the medial layer of the placental end of the umbilical artery of pre-eclamptic subjects.

Dopamine D_1 receptors located in the arterial smooth muscle mediate vasodilation. It is possible that the loss of this population of vasodilatory receptors may contribute to the increased resistance in the umbilical-placental circulation which occurs in pre-eclampsia.

Support from Italian National Research Council and "Tor Vergata" University are gratefully acknowledged.

Loss of dopamine D_2 receptors in the denervated rat kidney.

A.Rossodivita[1],M.H. Fernandes[2], A.Ricci[1], P.Soares-da-Silva[2] & F.Amenta[3].
[1]Dipto Scienze Cardiovascolari e Respiratorie Università "La Sapienza", Roma (Italy);
[2] Laboratorio de Farmacologia, Faculdade de Medicina do Porto (Portugal).
[3] Dipto di Sanità Pubblica e Biologia Cellulare, Università "Tor Vergata" Roma (Italy).

The influence of denervation on the density and pattern of dopamine D_2 receptors was investigated in male Wistar rats using combined radioligand binding and autoradiographic techniques. Unilateral renal denervation was performed by occluding the renal artery for 90 sec. This procedure caused a marked depletion of noradrenaline (NA) levels in the renal cortex and medulla without affecting dopamine (DA) concentrations. In fact, NA levels measured by HPLC with electrochemical detection averaged 1.10 ± 0.07 nmol/g in the non-denervated kidney and 0.03 ± 0.001 nmol/g in the denervated kidney. DA levels averaged 0.22 ± 0.002 nmol/g in the non-denervated kidney and 0.14 ± 0.001 nmol/g in the denervated kideny.

Radioligand binding experiments performed using ^{3}H-spiroperidol as a ligand revealed a dissociation constant value of 2.5 ± 0.2 nM in both control and denervated kidneys. The density of ^{3}H-spiroperidol binding sites was reduced by about 95% in denervated kidneys. Light microscopy autoradiography centered on the renal cortex revealed the development of silver grains which correspond to D_2 sites, in the proximal and distal convoluted tubules and no specific binding in the glomeruli. Denervation decreased the density of tubular D_2 sites by about 95%.

The above results collectively suggest that almost all tubular D_2 receptors in the rat renal cortex have a prejunctional localization.

Effects of long term L-DOPA treatment on diabetic nephropathy in the rat.

P. Mayer, M. Marthelmebs, C. Fontaine, D. Stephan,M. Grima & J.L. Imbs.
Institut de Pharmacologie, URA D0589 CNRS, Université Louis Pasteur et Service d' Hypertension Artérielle et Maladies Vasculaires, CHRU, 67000 Strasbourg, France.

The early stages of diabetic mellitus are characterized by glomerular hyperfiltration which may be involved in the progression of diabetic nephropathy. In a previous study (Marthelmebs et al. J. Cardiovasc. Pharmacol. 1991;18:243-253), we have shown that L-dopa, a precursor for endorenal DA synthesis, was able to correct the early glomerular hyperfiltration in streptozotocin-induced diabetic Wistar rats. In the present study, we followed the diabetic animals up to 14 months and compared the course of renal functions and albuminuria with and without L-dopa treatment.

Wistar rats received one injection of streptozotocin (60 mg/kg, i.v.); they were treated one week later with L-dopa (D-dopa) in the diet and were compared with untreated diabetic rats (D) and non diabetic rats (ND). At one month of evolution of the diabetes, "D-dopa" rats had no significant glomerular hyperfiltration (3.23 ± 0.13 vs 2.74 ± 0.18 ml/min, ND) in opposite to "D" rats 13.50 ± 0.33, $P< 0.05$). Microalbuminuria increased progressively from the tenth month of evolution in all diabetic rats but there was no difference in L-dopa treated rats (ND 1.9 ± 0.7; D, 9.1 ± 3.7; D-dopa, 8.3 ± 3.3 mg/day/100 g at 14 months of evolution; n =6-8).

Under constant daily L-dopa intake the urinary excretion of DA, as an index of endorenal DA synthesis, decreased progressively. The dose of L-dopa was therefore increased from 8 to 17 mg/day/100 g during the study.

Our results show that, despite early correction of glomerular hyperfiltration, L-dopa treatment was not able to avoid occurrence of microalbuminuria an early sign ot glomerular nephropathy. The reason for this escape from metabolism of L-dopa to DA or down regulation of the renal vascular DA receptors, is now under study.

Hormonal responses during insulin-mediated antinatriuresis in essential hypertension.

P. Coruzzi, A. Biggi, R. Ceriati, G. Mossini, N. Carra, L. Musiari, E. Bergamaschi* & A. Novarini.
Istituto di Semeiotica Medica & * Clinica Medica e Nefrologia, University of Parma, Italy.

Recent studies have implicated hyperinsulinemia as an etiologic factor in the development of essential hypertension; a sodium-retaining effect of insulin may have a role in promoting hypertension. In order to clarify the mechanisms responsible for carbohydrate-stimulated sodium retention, we examined the relation between sodium excretion, insulin secretion, urinary norepinephrine (NE) and dopamine (DA), PRA-aldosterone (PA) and prostaglandins activity in nine essential hypertensives undergoing extracellular fluid volume expansion by water inmersion (WI) alone and WI plus intravenous glucose load (IGTT) after an overnight fast.

Results of WI alone: there was a marked natriuretic event ($P<0.005$) a significant reduction of PRA and PA ($P<0.05$ and $P<0.01$, respectively), a significant increase of urinary 6-Keto PGF_{1alpha} ($P<0.01$) and a significant increase in both urinary NE and DA ($P<0.05$). Two weeks later, a WI study plus IGTT was performed in the same hypertensive subjects.

Results of WI plus IGTT: there was a blunted natriuretic event ($P<0.01$), the suppression of PRA and PA and the increase in both urinary NE and DA were similar to those obtained during WI alone, a significant reduction ($P=NS$) in urinary PGF_{1alpha} excretion was also found during WI plus IGTT; serum potassium did not change.

Our data suggest that an hyperinsulinemic state may mediate the antinatriuretic event found during WI plus IGTT in hypertensives either by a direct tubular effect (no changes in glomerular filtration rate) or by an insulin-mediated reduced prostaglandins activity.

Dopamine released from nerve endings activates presynaptic dopamine receptors in the human uterine artey.

T. R. A. Macedo, M. T. Morgadinho & C. A. Fontes Ribeiro.
Institute of Pharmacology and Experimental Therapeutics, Faculty of Medicine, University of Coimbra, Portugal.

Over the last years, some insight about the role of dopamine (DA) in peripheral tissues has been gained. However, only a few studies used human tissues and, on the other hand, the physiological role of the DA receptors is controversial. The purposes of the present study, carried out in human uterine arteries, were to determine: a) the presence of prejunctional DA receptors; b) a possible physiological role of these receptors in modulating sympathetic neurotransmission; c) the influence of alpha adrenergic and dopaminergic receptors upon catecholamine synthesis.

The preparations here previously submitted to a 30 min preincubation with 1 mM pargyline. Thereafter, the tissues were placed in perifusion chambers and washed out for 100 min with Krebs-Henseleit solution which contained 55 µM desoxycorticosterone and 7.5 µM cocaine; subsquently the fluid was continuously collected in 25 min samples. Two periods (Sl and S2) of electrical stimulauon (3 Hz, 1 msec, 100 V, 25 min) were performed. Yohimbine, sulpiride, SCH 23390 or apomorphine were added 30 min before S2. Catecholamine levels were determined by HPLC-ECD.

From these experiments it was concluded that DA represented about 6 % of the noradrenaline (NA) tissue content. The electrical stimuli released both DA and noradrenaline. However, the DA/NA ratio in the catecholamine overflow induced by nerve stimulation (S1) averaged 20%. Yohimbine (0.01-1 µM) significantly increased both DA and NA release. Sulpiride (0.1-1 µM) significantly increased the release of both amines. Apomorphine (1 µM) produced an opposite effect. Values of the Sl/S2 ratios were similar for both DA and noradrenaline. SCH 23390 did not significantly change catecholamine overflow. After yohimbine and sulpiride the tissue NA and DA content increased, an effect abolished by synthesis blockade.

These results suggest that in the human uterine artery DA and NA are co-released during electrical stimulation and activate presynaptic DA and alpha adrenergic receptors (auto-receptors), respectively, thereby playing a physiological control in transmitter release. These receptors may also influence catecholamine synthesis. Moreover, as the release of NA and DA is influenced at a similar extent by yohimbine and sulpiride, the amines probably co-exist in the same granular pool.

Carrier-mediated efflux of [^{3}H]-dopamine from the cat carotid body.

M. Pokorski, J. Albrecht & I. Fresko
Polish Academy of Sciences Medical Research Center, Warsaw, Poland.

Dopamine (DA) is released from the dense-cored vesicles of the carotid body (CB) chemoreceptor cells by natural and pharmacological stimuli. The dynamic events of DA release and their link to chemo-transduction are still unclear. In this study we tested to see if the nonvesicular, transport carrier-mediated efflux of DA could contribute to DA release in an in vitro CB. We looked for the evidence of the exchange/diffusion system in which the movement of externally present DA into a cell would stimulate the efflux of preloaded [^{3}H]-DA from that cell. We further evaluated the contribution of extracellular Na$^+$ to DA release by reducing the Na$^+$ concentration in the superfusion medium. Finally we evaluated the effects of the transport carrier blocker nomifensine on the [^{3}H]-DA efflux. CBs were excised from anesthetized cats, incubated with [^{3}H]-DA and placed on Whatman GF/B glass-fiber filters cut to fit a 25 mm Swinex filter unit. The filters were superfused with a Krebs-Henseleit medium and pulses of low sodium (50 mM Na$^+$ with choline replacement) or 1 mM DA, with and without nomifensine (1 μM), were applied. Radioactivity was counted in the eluates collected every 2 min. The pulse-induced [^{3}H]-DA efflux was expressed as % basal release. We found that both the unlabeled DA and low Na$^+$ pulses increased the efflux of preloaded [^{3}H]-DA; 1.4-fold and 2.5-fold, respectively. The low Na$^+$ overflow of [^{3}H]-DA was abolished by nomifensine which however did not affect the homoexchange of DA. These results suggest the existence of an Na$^+$-dependent carrier-mediated efflux of DA originating from a nonvesicular intracellular pool; a new finding with regard to the carotid body. The differential sensitivity of the nonvesicular DA release to a transport carrier blocker and the role of this release in chemotransduction require further studies.

Involvement of renal dopaminergic system in the control of vasoactive mediator release: Evidence for a functional D_2 receptor.

G. Durrieu, C. Damase-Michel, M.A. Tran, G. Bompart*, G. Tavernier, J.L. Montasturc & J.P. Girolami*.
Laboratoire de Pharmacologie Medicale et Clinique, INSERM U317, *INSERM U133, Faculte de Medecine,Toulouse, France.

A preponderance of data supports that renal tubular D_1 receptors control sodium excretion. However, there is yet no evidence associating renal D_2 binding sites with any functional response. Peripheral D_2 receptors are well known on postganglionic sympathetic nerves where they inhibit noradrenaline release. In contrast, their presence and function remain still discussed in renal cortex.

The aim of the present study was to investigate the involvement of the dopaminergic system in the control of the renal sympathetic tone. Thus, renal release of catecholamines was studied using incubation of dog renal cortical slices. This model permitted the study of the direct effects of selective D_1- and D_2-agonists such as fenoldopam and quinpirole on the renal catecholaminergic system in the absence of changes in perfusion pressure. Catecholamines (noradrenaline, adrenaline and dopamine) were measured by a sensitive HPLC method with electrochemical detection.

Addition of quinpirole (10^{-6} to 10^{-3} M) induced a dose-dependent decrease in noradrenaline and dopamine release from renal cortical slices which reached 59 % and 69 %, respectively, with 10^{-4} M quinpirole. Adrenaline release remained unchanged. By contrast, whatever the dose, fenoldopam failed to modify catecholamine release.

These data show that D_2 dopamine receptors activation inhibits noradrenaline release in isolated kidney cortical slices. They confirm the existence of such a renal D_2 receptor and suggest its potential involvement in the control of renal sympathetic tone.

Role of dopamine 1 and dopamine 2 receptors in the regulation of sodium excretion.

Ann-Christine Eklöf, Shanlin Chen & Anita Aperia.
Dept. of Paediatrics, Karolinska Institutet, S.t Görans Childrens Hospital, Stockholm, Sweden.

Dopamine (DA) produced in the kidney, acts as an autocrine and paracrine factor to inhibit tubular Na^+ reabsorption by inhibiting tubular Na^+, K^+-ATPase activity. In the proximal tubule Na^+,K^+-ATPase activity is inhibited by a synergistic action of D_1 and D_2 receptors. Yet several studies in man as well as in other species have shown that it is sufficient to administer the D_1 agonist, fenoldopam, to produce natriuresis and that inhibition of proximal tubular sodium reabsorption significantly contributes to this natriuresis. These apparently controversial observations have prompted us to study the interaction between endogenous dopamine and exogenously administered fenoldopam in rats.

The studies were performed on adult male Sprague-Dawley rats under euvolemic conditions. Fenoldopam 0.5 mg/kg/min significantly increased sodium excretion without altering the glomerular filtration rate. The simultaneous infusion of D_2 antagonist S-Sulperide 25 mg/kg/min completely abolished the natriuretic effect of fenoldopam. S-Sulperide alone had no effect on sodium excretion and glomerular filtration rate. It has been suggested that signals from D_2 receptors might interfere with the effects of norepinephrine which stimulates Na^+,K^+-ATPase activity and acts antinatriuretically. We therefore also determined the effects of the D_1 agonist and the D_2 antagonist on a denervated kidney. As expected, sodium excretion was higher in the denervated kidney than in the innervated kidney. The D_1 agonist did not further increase sodium excretion in the denervated kidney, while the D_2 antagonist caused a paradoxical increase of sodium excretion without altering the glomerular filtration rate. Conclusion: In the innervated kidney, dopamine causes natriuresis by interacting with both D_1 and D_2 receptors. D_2 receptor activation might abolish the effects of norepinephrine.

Characterization of the hypertensive profile in the nitric oxide-deprived rat: Prevention by L-arginine and reversibility by isosorbide 5-mononitrate.

A. Albino-Teixeira & P. Soares-da-Silva.
Dept. of Pharmacology & Therapeutics, Faculty of Medicine, 4200 Porto, Portugal.

Nitric oxide (NO) is believed to account for the actions of the endothelium-derived relaxing factor on vascular smooth muscle cells. Vascular endothelial cells synthetize NO from L-arginine by the action of a constitutive Ca^{++}-dependent NO-synthase as a transduction mechanism for the activation of the soluble guanylate cyclase in vascular smooth muscle. The acute administration of inhibitors of the NO-synthase results in vasoconstriction and systemic hypertension. The present study has evaluated the blood pressure profile during chronic administration of the NO-synthase inhibitor N^G-Nitro-L-arginine methyl esther (L-NAME) in drinking water as a NO-deprived rat hypertensive model. After a 7 day period of stabilization, normotensive male Wistar rats (n=10) were selected and given (L-NAME 5mg/100 ml) in drinking water. Control rats (n=10) were studied simultaneously for direct comparison of cardiovascular parameters. Blood pressure (systolic, SBP; diastolic, DBP) and heart rate were measured using a photoelectric tail cuff pulse detector; SBP and DBP was in normotensive rats, respectively, 106±2 and 78±2 mm Hg (n=10). The average water comsuption per animal was about 35 ml/day resulting in a mean intake of L-NAME of about 10 mg/kg. Twenty four hours after exposure to L-NAME, both SBP and DBP were found to be increased by 20 mm Hg; heart rate slightly decreased. During the next 13 days both SBP and DBP increased progressively reaching, respectively, 170±3 and 116±3 mm Hg. On day 14, six animals of either group were sacrificed and the heart, kidneys, liver, spleen, mesenteric and caudal arteries, brain stem, hypothalamus and parietal cortex were taken for determination of noradrenaline (NA) and dopamine (DA) content; blood from the renal vein was also collected and plasma concentrations of NA, adrenaline (AD) and dihydroxyphenylethylglycol (DOPEG) determined. Only in the left atrium of hypertensive rats was NA found to be increased (9.6±0.5 vs 6.4±0.5 nmol/g). NA concentrations in plasma were found to be increased in hypertensive rats, whereas AD DOPEG did not differ significantly between the two groups. Administration of the NO generating compound isosorbide 5-mononitrate (IS-5-MN; 20.4 mg/100 ml) in drinking water to L-NAME-treated rats resulted in a 25 mm Hg reduction of both SBP and DBP values; this dose of IS-5-MN did not change blood pressure values in control rats. L-arginine (100mg/100 ml) in drinking water was found unable to reduce SBP and DBP values in L-NAME-treated rats; however, previous administration of L-arginine (100 mg/100 ml) in drinking water completely prevented the hypertensive effect of L-NAME.

Supported by INIC (FmP1).

Renal formation and cellular transport of dopamine in the nitric oxide-deprived hypertensive rat.

P.Soares-da-Silva, M.H.Fernandes, M.Pestana, M.A.Vieira-Coelho & A.Albino-Teixeira.
Dept. of Pharmacology & Therapeutics, Faculty of Medicine, 4200 Porto, Portugal.

There is evidence suggesting that the renal formation of dopamine (DA) may be altered in some forms of hypertension, namely in salt-sensitive essential hypertensive subjects. The aim of the present work was to study the synthesis and cell outward transfer of DA in renal tissues of a new hypertensive model, the nitric-oxide deprived rat. The nitric-oxide deprived hypertensive rat was obtained by the administration to Wistar rats of N^G-Nitro-L-arginine methyl esther (L-NAME), the nitric oxide synthetase inhibitor, in drinking water (5mg/100 ml), as described elsewhere (1). Systolic and diastolic blood pressure was in normotensive control rats, respectively, 106 ± 1 and 74 ± 2 mm Hg, and in 14 days L-NAME-treated rats, respectively, 167 ± 2 and 116 ± 2 mm Hg. In some experiments, 14 days L-NAME+L-arginine (100 mg/100 ml) treated rats (normotensive) and hyperytensive animals to which L-NAME was given only for 7 days were used for the purposes of comparison. In some experiments, renal cortical slices were incubated for 15 min with increasing concentrations of L-DOPA (5 to 5000 μM) and the amounts of DA and of its deaminated metabolite DOPAC determined; DA and DOPAC levels were determined in both kidney slices and the incubation medium, in order to allow the determination of the fractional outflow of the two compounds. In other experiments, kidney homogenates were used and the kinetics of the enzyme aromatic L-amino acid decarboxylase (AAAD) determined. The formation of DA and DOPAC in kidney slices obtained from rats treated with L-NAME for 14 days was found to be twice that in either normotensive controls, rats treated with L-NAME+L-arginine (normotensive) or animals given L-NAME for 7 days (hypertensive). The kinetics (V_{max}, in nmol/mg protein/h; K_m, in μM) of the AAAD determined in kidney homogenates were as follows: controls (V_{max}=4.9$\pm$0.5; K_m=260$\pm$29), 14 days L-NAME (V_{max}=21.3$\pm$2.4; K_m=211$\pm$17), 14 days L-NAME+L-arginine (V_{max}= 5.7$\pm$0.5, K_m=298$\pm$32) and 7 days L-NAME (V_{max}=4.6$\pm$0.5; K_m=231$\pm$27). The outward cell transfer of DA was found to be similar in either experimental group of animals; the V_{max} and the K_m values for the saturable component were, respectively, 343 nmol/g/15 min and 586 nmol. The urinary excretion of DA was also found to be significantly increased in the last 5 days of the 14 days L-NAME administration. The results presented suggest that the increased renal formation of DA in the nitric-oxide deprived hypertensive rat may correspond to a compensatory mechanism.

(1) Albino-Teixeira A & Soares-da-Silva P (this volume).

Supported by INIC (FmP1).

Renal dopamine excretion and vasodilatation in spontaneously hypertensive rats (SHR).

M. Barthelmebs, C. Fontaine, M. Grima, D. Stephan & J. L. Imbs.
Institut de Pharmacologie, URA D0589 CNRS, Université Louis Pasteur et Service d'Hypertension Arterielle et Maladies Vasculaires, CHRU, 67000 Strasbourg, France.

Endorenal dopamine (DA) synthesis and DA-induced vasodilatation were evaluated in SHR and age-matched normotensive WKY rats. The renal DA excretion was measured in a 24 h urine collection (free DA, HPLC with electrochemical detection) under basal conditions and after L-dopa administration (10 mg/kg sc).

In 7 week-old rats, the sodium excretion was lower in SHR but the basal urinary DA excretion was increased (*$P<0.05$); L-dopa-stimulated DA excretion was identical in SHR and WKY rats. In 12 week-old rats, the sodium excretion became similar but the basal DA excretion remained enhanced in SHR.

mean±SEM (n=12)		SysBP (mm Hg)	UVNa-basal (mmol/day)	UVDA-basal (nmol/day)	UVDA-dopa (μmol/day)
7 weeks	WKY	117±3	1.8±0.1	6±2	2.05±0.67
	SHR	145±5*	1.4±0.1*	16±4*	2.03±0.53
12 weeks	WKY	125±3	1.5±0.1	6±1	1.84±0.43
	SHR	190±3*	1.7±0.1	10±1*	1.36±0.15

The renal vasodilatory effect of DA was controlled in isolated perfused kidneys taken from 12 week-old SHR and WKY rats in the presence of alpha- and beta-adrenoceptor blocking drugs and after the basal renal vascular tone had been restored by PGF_{2alpha}. DA induced a similar renal relaxation in SHR and WKY rats (EC_{50}=0.7±0.1 and 1.7±0.4 μmol/1; E_{max}=100±2 and 91±5% relaxation on PGF_{2alpha}-induced renal vascular tone, n=5).

These results show that renal extraneuronal DA synthesis (as reflected by urinary DA excretion) is enhanced during the development ot hypertension in SHR. Despite normal renal DA vascular effects, established hypertension occurred in these animals. Abnormal renal sodium handling in the proximal tubule may be involved.

Antihypertensive effect of TA-870, a novel dopamine prodrug, in spontaneously hypertensive rat.

Kiyonobu Tanaka, Shuichi Shigetomi & Soitu Fukuchi
The Third Dept. Internal Medicine, Fukushima Medical College, Fukushima-City, JAPAN 960-12

Objectives: In the present study, we tried to demonstrate the effect of N-(N-acetyl-L-methionyl)-3,4-bis(ethoxycarbonyl)dopamine, a novel dopamine prodrug (Docarpamine, TA-870), on blood pressure, heart rate and regional contents of dopamine and its metabolites in the peripheral tissues of spontaneously hypertensive rats (SHR).

Methods: Ten male SHR and 9 male wistar-Kyoto rats (WKY), aged 9~12 weeks, were used in this study. Their left femoral veins for the drug injection and left femoral arteries for monitoring mean arterial blood pressure (MDP) and heart rate (HR) were cannulated under intraperitoneal anesthesia by pentobarbital sodium salt. Following the administration of either TA-870 (200 µg/kg) or vehicle, MBP and HR were continously monitored for 45 min. In the second series of the study, rats were killed by decapitation 20 min after the injection and brain tissues (hypothalamus, striatum and medulla oblongata) and peripheral tissues [lung, liver, kidney (cortex and medulla) and adrenal gland] were removed for the determination of tissue contents of dopamine and its metabolites (DOPAC, HVA and 3-methoxytyramine), norepinephrine (NE) and epinephrine (E) by HPLC with electrochemical detection.

Results: TA-870 induced a significant decrease of MDP (before: 194.3±23.5 mmHg and 20 min after: 165.6±9.8 mmHg, P<0.025) following a slight initial increase, but there was no significant change in MBP in WKY. The maximal depressor effect of TA-870 was observed 20 min after the injection and recovered to the basal level 40 min after the injection. In SHR unlike in WKY, TA-870 decreased HR (before: 282.8±20.6 beats/min and 20 min after: 257.5±26.1 beats/min), and this decrease in HR was positively correlated to the decrease in MBP (r=0.926, p<0.005). In renal cortex and medulla of both SHR and WKY, contents of dopamine and HVA markedly increased (2~5 fold) following TA-870 injection. TA-870 increased all fractions of catecholamine in adrenal gland in WKY, while there was a slight decrease in the contents of NE and E in SHR. The change of brain contents of dopamine and its metabolites by TA-870 was slight and insignificant.

Conclusion: This is the first report demonstrating that TA-870 has a BP decreasing effect in SHR, probably due to the peripheral action of dopamine resulting in the suppression of NE release and/or the inhibition of tyrosine hydroxylase in the sympathoadrenal system.

FPL 65447AA: A selective D_1-receptor agonist.

G. W. Smith, M. I. Christie, * F. Ince, A. K. Nicol, * B. Springthorpe, G. E. Williams &
A. Verity.
Fisons plc, Pharmaceutical Division, Research and Development Laboratories,
Departments of Pharmacoiogy and * Medicinal Chemistry, Loughborough,
Leicestershire, LE11 ORH,UK.

FPL 65447AA was assessed both for agonist activity at the various receptors
stimulated by dopamine and for cardiovascular activity using methods described
previously (Brown et al., 1985a and 1985b).

FPL 65447AA injected directly into the
anaesthetised dog renal artery increased renal
blood flow (blocked by SCH 23390) by
reducing renal vascular resistance, with a
potency 1.3±0.2 (n=6) times that of dopamine.
In the rabbit ear artery (D_2) and in the guinea-
pig atria ($ß_1$), trachea ($ß_2$) and aorta (alpha $_1$),
no agonism was demonstrated at up to 100
µM. In contrast to dopamine, FPL 65447AA
was only a weak postjunctional alpha$_2$ agonist
(antagonised by 1 µM rauwolscine) in the
rabbit saphenous vein, pretreated with 1 µM
prazosin, with a potency 17 times weaker than
dopamine (n=12).

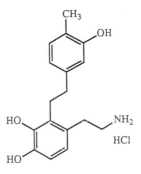

FPL 65447AA infusion (1-10 $\mu g.kg^{-1}.min^{-1}$, i.v. each for 30 min) was examined in
12 anaesthetised dogs. It produced a dose-related (responses at highest infusion)
increase in renal (16±2 %, n=6) and superior mesenteric (15±3 %, n=6) blood flows
associated with a fall in renal (26±2%) and mesenteric (25±3 %) vascular resistances.
Blood pressure was reduced (15±2 %, n=12) whilst heart rate and contractility were
only slightly reduced (9±1 % and 8±1 %, respectively, n=12). With the exception of the
cardiac responses, SCH 23390 infusion antagonised the effects of FPL 65447AA.

It is concluded that by acting as a selective agonist at the peripheral D_1-receptor,
FPL 65447AA results in an increase in blood flow in the kidney and gut.

Brown R. A., et al. (1985a). Br. J. Pharmacol., 85: 599-608.
Brown R. A., et al. (1985b). Br. J. Pharmacol., 85: 609-619.

ABBOTT-68930: An orally active D_1 agonist in the conscious dog.

M. I. Christie & G. W. Smith.
Fisons plc, Pharmaceutical Division, Department of Pharmacology, Cardiovascular Section, Loughborough, Leicestershire, LE11 ORH, UK.

The effects of the D_1 agonist A-68930 (DeNinno et al., 1991) were studied in conscious dogs chronically implanted with a Data Sciences blood pressure monitor in the right femoral artery and a pulsed doppler flow probe on the left renal artery, a model similiar to that previously described (Smith et al., 1990).

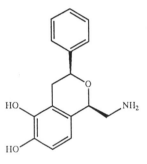

Infusion of A-68930 (0.03-1 nmol.kg^{-1}.min^{-1}, i.v., n=4) or fenoldopam (0.1-3 nmol.kg^{-1}.min^{-1}, n=6) produced a dose-related fall in renal vascular resistance (RVR) and a rise in renal blood flow (RBF), together with a dose-related hypotension and tachycardia. No behavioural changes were seen. On the basis of the increase in RBF, A-68930 (geometric mean ED_{20} of 0.068, range 0.043-0.110 nmol.kg^{-1}.min^{-1}) was calculated to be 6.9 times more potent than fenoldopam. At the end of a sub-maximal infusion, the RBF effects of A-68930 declined with a significantly longer half-time than fenoldopam (15.4 ± 1.7 vs 3.5 ± 0.5 minutes, P< 0.01).

Oral administration of A-68930 (0.03-01 µmol.kg^{-1}) or fenoldopam (1-10 µmol.kg^{-1}) also produced a dose-related fall in RVR and an increase in RBF with hypotension and tachycardia. Using the peak RBF changes produced by oral dosing, A-68930 (mean ED_{20} of 2.6, range 1.6-4.0 nmol.kg^{-1}) was calculated to be 660 times more potent than fenoldopam (n=3). Furthermore the RBF effects of oral A-68930 took longer to recover to baseline (5-6 hours than an equi-effective dose of fenoldopam (1-2 hours). In two dogs, the oral effects of A-68930 were attenuated by concommitant i.v. infusion of SCH 23390 (10 µg.kg^{-1} + 15 µg.kg^{-1}.hr^{-1}), confirming an action at the D_1 receptor.

These data indicate that A-68930 is a potent, orally active D_1 agonist with a longer duration of action than fenoldopam. The increased potency of A-68930 after oral dosing suggests that it is either better absorbed than fenoldopam or less susceptible to first pass metabolism.

Smith, G. W., et al. (1990) Br. J. Pharmacol., 100: 295-300.
DeNinno, M. P., et al . (1991) J. Med. Chem., 34. 2561-2569.

Effect of epinine on systemic hemodynamics and regional blood flows in conscious pigs.

L.J. van Woerkens[1], A. J. Man in 't Veld[2], W.J. van der Giessen[1], F. Boomsma[2] & P.D. Verdouw [1].
Laboratory for Experimental Cardiology, Thoraxcenter[1] and Dept. of Internal Medicine I [2], Erasmus University Rotterdam, P.0. Box 1738, 3000 DR Roterdam, The Netherlands.

Intravenous infusions (1, 2.5, 5 and 10 µg/kg/min for 10 min) were used to evaluate the cardiovascular effects of epinine (N-methyl-dopamine) (EP) in 8 conscious pigs. EP is a non-selective and non-specific dopamine (DA) agonist, that also stimulates alpha and beta-adrenoceptors. EP (1-5 µg/kg/min) increased cardiac output up to 15±5% (P<0.05), due to an increase in heart rate (24±6%), but an increase in stroke volume (16±4%) caused the further increase in cardiac output at 10 µg/kg/min. Mean arterial blood pressure decreased gradually from 100±5 mmHg to 84±4 mmHg, but increased to 89±4 mmHg during infusion of 10 µg/kg/min (P<0.05). Systemic vascular resistance decreased after infusion of 5 µg/kg/min, but did not change further during the highest dose. LV dP/dt_{max} increased only at 10 µg/kg/min. Myocardial blood flow did not change at any dose. Flow to adrenals and spleen increased dose-dependently, but decreased to stomach and skin, while flow to the kidneys, liver, small intestine and skeletal muscle did not change. Cerebral blood flow increased only at the highest dose. Further studies are needed to evaluate the contribution of activation of DA and β_2-adrenoceptors to the EP-induced vasodilation of the various regional vascular beds.

Renal effects of dopamine, dobutamine and dopexamine: significance of dopaminergic stimulation during similar increases in cardiac output.

N.V. Olsen, J. Lund, P.F. Jensen, K. Espersen, I.L. & Kanstrup.
Departments of Anaesthesia and Clinical Physiology, Herlev Hospital, University of Copenhagen, DK-2730 Herlev, Denmark.

Overall renal effects of low-dose dopamine (DA) was compared to the effects of dobutamine (DB), which stimulates adrenergic β_1 but not DA receptors, and dopexamine (DX), which predominantly acts via adrenergic β_2 and D_1 receptors. Each drug was randomly given for 2 h on three different occasions to eight normal subjects in doses adjusted to produce a similar increase in cardiac output (CO). CO increased 33% (DA, $P<0.001$), 35% (DB, $P<0.01$) and 30% (DX, $P<0.01$), respectively. Doses (mean±SD) of DA, DB and DX were 2.90±0.19, 4.92±0.40 and 1.00±0.02 µg/kg/min, respectively. Mean arterial pressure increased by 16% ($P<0.05$) during DB, but remained unchanged during DA and DX. DA and DX increased effective renal plasma flow (ERPF) by 22% ($P<0.001$) and 14% ($P<0.001$), respectively, whereas ERPF remained unchanged during DB. The increase in ERPF was smaller during DX compared to DA ($P<0.05$). All 3 drugs only caused small, insignificant increases in GFR. Lithium elearance (C_{Li}) which was used to estimate proximal tubular outflow, increased by 37% ($P<0.001$) and 32% ($P<0.001$) during DA and DX, but was not changed by DB. Calculated absoluts proximal reabsorption rate (APR=GFR-C_{Li}) decreased by 16% ($P<0.05$) during DA, but remained unchanged during DB and DX. DA increased sodium clearance (C_{Na}) by 108% ($P<0.01$), but the increase during DX (58%) was not significant. DB tended to decrease C_{Na}. The finding that DA and DX in contrast to DB significantly increased ERPF with similar increases in CO is consistent with a specific, vasodilating effect of DA and DX on renal vasculature secondary to stimulation of renal DA receptors. Only DA significantly increased C_{Na}, and the decrease in APR suggests that a direct effect on proximal tubular reabsorption contributed to the DA-induced natriuresis.

© 1993 Pergamon Press Ltd.
Printed in Great Britain.

Increase in plasma dopamine by contaminated tyramine.

A.H. vd Meiracker, F. Boomsma, A.J. Man in `t Veld & M.A.D.H. Schalekamp.
Dept. of Internal Medicine I, University Hospital Dijkzigt, Erasmus University,
Rotterdam, The Netherlands.

The existence of peripheral dopaminergic nervous system in man as a possible source of plasma dopamine (DA) is still debated. Standard tests such as tilting, exercise or cold provocation invariably cause an increase in plasma noradrenaline (NA) but not in DA. In attempt to find evidence for the existence of a peripheral dopaminergic nervous system in man the effect of graded i.v. infusions of tyramine hydrochloride (TyrHCl) (5, 10 and 15 µg/kg/min for 10 minutes) on arterial (a) and venous (v) levels of NA and DA were studied in healthy volunteers. TyrHCl was infused via a cannula in a forearm vein. Blood was sampled via cannula's located in the antecubital vein and brachial artery of the contralateral arm. Infusion of TyrHCl (Merck) in 5 subjects caused dose-dependent increases in plasma NA and DA. With the highest dose of tyramine baseline NAa rose from 167±65 (mean±SD) to 320±72 pg/ml and NAv from 183±78 to 306±78 pg/ml, whereas DAa rose from 17±9 to 66±28 and DAv from 15±7 to 36±11 pg/ml. In all 5 subjects the increase in DAa was higher than the increase in DAv indicating that there was no net production of DA in the arm. Explanations for the preferential increase in DAa could be TyrHCl-induced release of DA somewhere else in the body and/or contamination of TyrHCl with DA. Analysis of infused TyrHCl revealed that it contained minute amounts of DA (300 pg DA per µg TyrHCl, but no detectable NA). When the TyrHCl solution was shaken vigorously with alumina at pH 8.6 for 4 min, more than 97 % of the DA was removed. During infusion of this purified TyrHCl in 2 other subjects baseline NAa rose from respectively 186 and 119 to 326 and 272 pg/ml with the highest dose and baseline NAv from, respectively, 186 and 145 to 298 and 286 pg/ml while baseline DAa and DAv did not change. Newly obtained batches of TyrHCl from various supplies (Merck, Sigma, Fluka, Aldrich, BDH,Serva) also contained DA (respectively 90,30,5,30,100, and 60 pg DA per µg TyrHCl. In conclusion, the existence of a peripheral dopaminergic nervous system which releases DA into the circulation during TyrHCl stimulation is not supported by our findings. Moreover, investigators should be aware that commercially available TyrHCl contains DA in variable amounts.

Differential cardiovascular and neuroendocrine effects of epinine and dopamine in conscious pigs before and after adrenoceptor blockade.

L.J. van Woerkens[1] , A. J. Man in 't Veld[2], W J. van der Giessen[1] , F.Boomsma[2] & P.D. Verdouw[1].
Laboratory for Experimental Cardiology, Thoraxcenter[1] and Dept. of Internal Medicine I [2], Erasmus University Rotterdam, P.0. Box 1738, 3000 DR Rotterdam, The Netherlands.

Effects of epinine (EP) or dopamine (DA) (1-10 µg/kg/min) on hemodynamics, catecholamines and prolactin (PRL) were studied in conscious pigs. EP increased cardiac output (CO, $24\pm6\%$) and heart rate (HR) at infusion rates < 10 µg/kg/min. At 10 µg/kg/min, HR decreased slightly ($10\pm3\%$) and stroke volume increased (15%, $P<0.05$). Mean arterial pressure (MAP) decreased (< 5 µg/kg/min), but increased by 4.0 ± 1.8 mmHg during infusion of 10 µg/kg/min. Systemic vascular resistance (SVR) decreased ($23\pm3\%$, < 10 µg/kg/min). LVdP/dt$_{max}$ increased during the two highest infusion rates ($22\pm6\%$, $P<0.05$). After the infusion was stopped there was an abrupt increase in HR ($18\pm4\%$, $P<0.05$) and a further decrease in SVR. Adrenoceptor blockade (alpha and beta BL) inhibited all EP-induced changes. DA caused similar increases in CO ($27\pm3\%$) as EP, the only difference being that HR continued to increase ($32\pm5\%$) while MAP ($13\pm3\%$) and SVR continued to decrease ($31\pm3\%$). Alpha, betaBL did not affect the DA-induced changes in CO, SVR and MAP, but attenuated the increases in HR and LVdP/dt$_{max}$. Norepinephrine (NE) and epinephrine (E) did not change during infusion of EP or DA, but NE increased by 50% after stopping EP. After alpha BL NE and E did not change during DA, which contrasted with a decrease ot $55\pm5\%$ ($P<0.05$) in NE during EP. PRL decreased from 480 ± 40 to 270 ± 50 pg/ml (P < 005) during EP, but did not change during DA. The effects of EP and DA on MAP ,SVR, NE and PRL show that in conscious pigs, EP is more potent alpha, beta$_2$ and D$_2$ agonist, but a weaker D$_1$ agonist than DA.

Metabolism and pharmacology of dopamine prodrug docarpamine (TA-870).

Shinsuke Nishiyama, Masayoshi Yoshikawa & Isao Yamaguchi.
Tanabe Seiyaku Co., Ltd., Toda, Japan.

Docarpamine, N-(N-acetyl-L-methionyl)-3,4-bis (ethoxycarbonyl) dopamine, is an orally available dopamine prodrug. Docarpamine is hydrolyzed to dopamine via deethoxycarbonyl docarpamine (DECD). In a first-pass metabolism study in anesthetized dogs, a part of intraduodenal dose of docarpamine (30 mg/kg) was converted to DECD in the small intestinal wall, and remaining unchanged docarpamine was almost completely hydrolyzed to DECD in the liver. DECD was hydrolyzed to free-dopamine largely in the liver during circulation. When equimolar doses of docarpamine and dopamine hydrochloride were administered orally to dogs, docarpamine elevated plasma free-dopamine to much higher concentrations than dopamine hydrochloride. Renal blood flow was increased in correlation with the augmented levels of free-dopamine. Docarpamine also increased cardiac contractility and output in anesthetized dogs. The renal and cardiac effects of docarpamine were inhibited by D_1 and ß antagonists, respectively. On the other hand, docarpamine and DECD had no effect on D_1, alpha and $ß_1$ receptors in vitro. Docarpamine showed much weaker vomiting effect than levodopa in dogs and had no effect on the CNS in mice and rats.

These effects show that docarpamine is an orally available dopamine prodrug selective for peripheral organs.

Rapid break-down of dopamine in pig plasma.

F. Boomsma, L.J. van Woerkens*, A.J. Man in 't Veld, P.D. Verdouw* & M.A.D.H. Schalekamp.
Departments of Internal Medicine I and Experimental Cardiology*, Erasmus University / University Hospital Dijkzigt, Dr. Molewaterplein 40, 3015 GD Rotterdam, The Netherlands.

Infusions of dopamine (DA) and epinine (EPI) in pigs showed that measured plasma concentrations of DA were quite variable, due to a rapid break-down of DA, but not of EPI. Plasma had been prepared from blood collected into chilled 10-ml heparinized tubes containing 12 mg of glutathione; after centrifugation plasma had been separated and frozen at -70°C until assayed by HPLC with electrochemical or fluorimetric detection. Under these conditions catecholamines, including DA, are quile stable in human plasma.

When known amounts of norepinephrine (NE), epinephrine (E), DA and EPI were added to pig plasma, and recovery was determined after various times (1 ,2,3 and 4 h) at 20° or 4°C, indeed recoveries of NE, E and EPI were excellent, but not those of DA. After 4 h at 20°C all DA had disappeared, while after 4 h at 4°C recovery was 50%. In human plasma recoveries of all catecholamines including DA were >92%. Attempts to prevent the break-down of DA by adding more glutathione (10 mg/ml) or pargyline, clorgyline, EDTA, sodium bisulphite (all 10 mg/ml) or combinations of these were all unsuccessful, as long as the pH of the plasma was kept unchanged at ± 7.8. Lowering the pH of the plasma proved to be successful: however, when the plasma was acidified with 50 or 100 µl of 1 N HCl per ml (respectively, resulting in pH 5 and 3) recovery of DA after 4 h at 20°C was, respectively, 96% and 100%, the same as of NE, E and EPI.

The surprising selective break-down of DA in pig plasma suggests that large inter-species differences may exist regarding stability of catecholamines in plasma. In each species stability should be established separately by recovery experiments.

The nature of the break down product of DA in pig plasma, and of the responsible agent (probably an enzyme) is currently under investigation.

Pharmacokinetics and -dynamics of ibopamine in autonomic failure.

A.H. vd Meiracker, F. Boomsma,W. Rensma, A.J. Man in 't Veld & M.A.D.H. Schalekamp.
Dept. Internal Medicine I, University Hospital Dijkzigt, Rotterdam, The Netherlands.

Introduction: Ibopamine (IBO) is a new, orally active, dopaminergic agent. After oral administration IBO is rapidly hydrolyzed to its active compound epinine (EPI). Free (F) EPI is subject to substantial first-pass sulphate conjugation. Since, in addition to its dopaminergic activity, EPI has agonistic activity for alpha- and ß-adrenoceptors, we explored the effect of IBO on postural hypotension in pure autonomic failure (PAF). Protocol: In 3 patients with PAF (patient A, male, age 72 years,norepinephrine (NA) 55 pg/ml; patient B, female, age 32 years, NA 9 pg/ml; patient C, female, age 42 years, NA 2 pg/ml) 60° passive head-up tilting (HUT) for 10 min was performed before and after an oral dose of IBO of 100 mg. In patient B, this procedure was repeated after a 2nd dose of IBO, because no response occurred to the 1 st dose. Mean arterial pressure (MAP) was measured in the radial artery and heart rate (HR) was derived from the ECG. Plasma levels of F and conjugated (CON) EPI after IBO were determined at 10 min intervals. Results: Peak levels of F EPI were observed 10 (patients B and C) and 30 min (patient A) after oral administration of IBO. Peak levels of F and CON EPI were respectively 4.5 and 16.5 ng/l in patient A, 0.2 and 6.3 ng/l after the lst dose and 2.8 and 151 ng/l after the 2nd dose in patient B, and 29.8 and 67.8 ng/l in patient C. The variations in F EPI were reflected in the hemodynamic responses. In response to HUT fall in MAP was diminished by 20 mmHg in patient A, 30 min after IBO, and by 18 mmHg in patient B, 10 min after IBO (2nd dose), whereas after 30 min no hemodynamic effect was observed anymore. The extremely high levels of F EPI in patient C were associated with severe hypertension and tachycardia (maximal increments in MAP and HR of respectively 42 mmHg and 56 bpm) and improvement of postural hypotension persisted for 40 min. Conclusion: IBO improves postural hypotension in patients with PAF. However, in light of its observed highly variable intra- and inter-individual pharmacokinetics, more pharmacokinetic and -dynamic studies are needed before it can be advocated for this disorder.

AUTHOR INDEX

SUBJECT INDEX

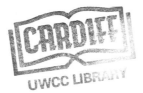